'The eloquent and poetic language of the classics of Chinese medicine has always seemed incommensurable with modern Western scientific medicine. No longer. Dr Keown provides clear and compelling evidence that both systems are describing the same processes in the human body. Some kind of synthesis is now in prospect, and the implications are enormous.'

– John Hamwee, acupuncturist and author of
Acupuncture for New Practitioners

'It is surprising how little research has been done over the years to examine the relationship of acupuncture to Western medicine. Now at last we have Dr Keown's thoughtful and stimulating book to help fill this gap. Dr Keown talks from personal experience of working on both sides of this medical divide. His book is an invaluable contribution to helping practitioners of both disciplines understand how far they speak a common medical language, though they may express themselves in somewhat different terms.'

– Nora Franglen, Founder of the School of Five Element
Acupuncture (SOFEA) and author of The Handbook of Five
Element Practice, Keepers of the Soul, Patterns of Practice
and The Simple Guide to Five Element Acupuncture

'Unusually for a doctor, Daniel Keown has a deep knowledge of the theories and practice of acupuncture and Chinese medicine. His obvious love and profound understanding of anatomy and physiology means that he is almost uniquely qualified to explain how acupuncture "works" according to the paradigm of modern science. This is an important book and essential reading for anyone interested in bridging the gap in understanding between Chinese medicine and conventional medical science.'

– Peter Mole, Dean of the College of Integrated
Chinese Medicine, Reading, UK and author of
Acupuncture for Body, Mind and Spirit

D1292496

'I started reading this book and thought "wow!" – I couldn't put it down! Daniel Keown is both a Western medical doctor and an Acupuncturist. Using his engaging writing style he makes sense of how the latest scientific understanding of systems theory unites with the holism of our oldest medical tradition. Everyone from the general public to Western and Eastern medical practitioners – in fact, anyone who is curious about the remarkable way the human body functions and develops – should read this book.'

– Angela Hicks, Joint Principal of the College of Integrated Chinese Medicine, Reading, UK, and author of The Principles of Chinese Medicine

The Spark *in the* Machine

How the Science of Acupuncture Explains the Mysteries of Western Medicine

DR DANIEL KEOWN M.B. CH.B., LIC. AC.

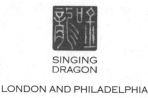

SINGING
DRAGON

LONDON AND PHILADELPHIA

Publisher's note
This book does not attempt to map Chinese medicine onto Western medicine, but explores how the body is better understood through a synthesis of both paradigms.

First published in 2014
by Singing Dragon
an imprint of Jessica Kingsley Publishers
73 Collier Street
London N1 9BE, UK
and
400 Market Street, Suite 400
Philadelphia, PA 19106, USA

www.singingdragon.com

Library of Congress Cataloging in Publication Data
Keown, Daniel.
  The spark in the machine : how the science of Acupuncture
explains the mysteries of western medicine
/ Dr. Daniel Keown, M.B. Ch, B. Lic. Ac.
     pages cm
  Includes bibliographical references.
  ISBN 978-1-84819-196-9 (alk. paper)
  1. Acupuncture. 2. Integrative medicine. 3. Medicine, Chinese. I. Title.
  RM184.K38 2014
  615.8'92--dc23
                         2013037291

British Library Cataloguing in Publication Data
A CIP catalogue record for this book is available from the British Library

ISBN 978 1 84819 196 9
eISBN 978 0 85701 154 1

Printed and bound in the United States

To Denis, my father, ace surgeon and man of God, who taught me about fascia with a Sainsbury's bag; and Margaret, my mother, who taught me that Art comes from the Heart…

ACKNOWLEDGEMENTS

I will always owe an enormous debt of gratitude to the irrepressible Alexandra Hain-Cole, without whose patient guidance into the World of Grammar this book may never have been borne.

There are too many people to thank, but special thanks to the (probably drug-addled) burglar who returned my drawings; Dr Ironside for bullying me into writing this book; Ranald MacDonald for showing me the art of Chinese medicine and Dr Mike Roberts for the art of Western; Manchester Medical School and the College of Integrated Chinese Medicine for their wisdom and patience; James Cole for his words and inventing a new profession – lexiconsultant; and Jessica Kingsley, Victoria and Octavia for their clarity of vision.

Lastly, to my wife, the beautiful Josephine, who has not only borne me a wonderfully naughty little boy Harrison and a gorgeous little girl Cora, but also my hopes and crazy dreams. This book is your book too, my love.

PREFACE

It was whilst studying in China with probably one of the most respected Acupuncturists in the world – Dr Wang Ju-Yi – that the embryo of this book was first conceived. Dr Wang chose his words with the studied patience of a man who has spent most of his 70 years thinking deeply about the mysteries of Acupuncture.* The very beautiful and wonderfully modest assistant Mei then translated his words before I could start to understand anything. In turn I would then nod, sometimes in understanding, but often, probably, vaguely idiotically.

Dr Wang understood it was the spaces in the body where Acupuncture acted, and when he spoke of its relationships I found myself realising that his deep understanding of Acupuncture shared much with embryological science. I was excited by this, for once I felt I had something interesting to tell *him*: was he aware of this, the parallels between embryology and Chinese Acupuncture channels?

Dr Ju-Yi thought about it for a while and then, speaking with his characteristic slow steady rhythm but with an added glint in his eye said: 'No…but you must go and write a book on it.'

This is that book. It is to be read and enjoyed by anyone with an interest in how our amazing bodies are formed. It is a book that weaves together the very latest in our modern understanding of embryology and the very oldest of medical traditions. I hope in some way it enlightens your knowledge of the body and furthers your understanding of the most complete medical tradition in the world.

---

* You may have noticed the 'A' of 'Acupuncture' is capitalised. The convention when writing about Chinese medicine is that concepts and organs (such as 'Kidney') are capitalised to distinguish them from the Western medical physical counterparts (a difference which mainly disappears when explored deeper, as explained in Parts II and III).

CONTENTS

Why Can't Humans Regenerate?

When I was three years old I caught my thumb in a folding chair. I cannot remember this episode, filled as it must have been with blood and pain, but my mother does. She packed the amputated tip of the thumb on ice and rushed me to the Emergency Department, where a surgeon sewed it back on again. I still have the scar on my thumb now, running parallel to the base of my nail.

What my mother didn't know, and what most doctors still don't, is that my thumb would almost certainly have grown back perfectly without any treatment. It would have regenerated in the same way as some amphibians can grow back their tails or legs. Bone, nail, nerves, blood vessels, the whole lot. All it needed was a gentle clean, a non-adherent dressing, and a lollipop to soothe my frayed, three-year-old nerves.

It turns out humans *can* regenerate, but only the very tips of their fingers and only children, who still have strong Qi (we'll come to this). In the 1970s a Sheffield paediatrician even published a paper on this effect in the *Journal of Paediatric Surgery*.[1] Her results were unequivocal: amputations above the last joint in children under six left to heal naturally would regrow, the entire finger, without a scar or deformity!

It is somewhat amazing that this fact is so little known in the medical community. Having worked in the Emergency Department for ten years I have only ever met one colleague who was aware of this fact, despite the implications it has for patient care. The reason for this to me is clear: it strikes at the core of what we think we know about medicine. If people can regenerate fingers then how do they do so, and what else can they regenerate? Medical schools would have to open up a new department.

The research into regeneration in humans is so slim that I have only ever seen one book on it, yet it is at the heart of the healing principle.[2] An orthopaedic surgeon in America, R.O. Becker, spent decades looking into the ability of salamanders to regenerate. His interest was in the non-union of bone fractures, literally a crippling problem that can occur for no clear reason. His findings led to medically approved devices for using electricity to cure 'non-unions', but it was these findings themselves that were most amazing.

Becker chose salamanders to experiment on because of their ability to regrow limbs, but he could have used any number of primitive animals that regenerate. Salamanders never suffer from non-union of broken bones for, even if they have no limb left to reunite, they can just grow a new one. Although salamanders are amphibians, their legs are functionally very similar to ours. They have bones, joints, nerves, blood vessels, and muscles, tendons and ligaments. In fact, they have everything we have in our legs, just smaller and covered in green skin.

A salamander that has had its leg removed will make a stumpy blood clot at the end and then over the course of the next few weeks it will grow a shiny new green leg. It's amphibian magic!

Becker was intrigued by this power. After some research, he started to measure the electrical currents that would occur at the site of injury after amputating his salamanders' legs. He had already noticed that there was a tiny electrical gradient from the salamander's head to fingers (if that is what a salamander has). He noticed that this current was so small that it was almost unmeasurable. It was in micro-amperes, but was consistent and was consistently more negative at the head. What he found was that after he amputated the limb there was a reversal in the polarity of the normal electrical current and that this reversal would cause the limb regeneration.

Most students of medicine will not find anything unusual about animals generating electricity. Nerves are constantly able to produce this and some animals can even generate large electric shocks. What was unusual about this electricity was that it was a DC current. Nerve electricity is AC – it has an up and down, like the power from the mains. The current Becker was measuring was constant, like that from a battery.

Now, it would be nice to say at this point that no animals were harmed in these experiments, but that is clearly not true… What is incredible, though, is that at the end of the experiments it *appeared* that no animals had been harmed! Regeneration is a truly miraculous event.

What Becker found is that this reversal of electrical current would cause changes in the salamanders' blood cells in the region of injury. They would de-differentiate (differentiation is the process of stem cells turning into specialised cells such as muscles). In other words, the red blood cells would wind back the embryological clock, unlocking their DNA until they were primitive stem cells again. Then they would start rebuilding the limb from scratch, differentiating into bone, nerve, muscle, whatever was needed. Within a few weeks the job was done and the salamander was back on four legs again. So long as the salamander had enough food, this could be repeated many times.

Any student of medicine may have spotted a deliberate mistake in the above: red blood cells don't have DNA in them; they have no nucleus. Indeed, this is true, red cells have no nucleus in humans, but in more primitive animals red cells *are* nucleated. They have all the genetic code present: large parts have been turned off to enable the cell to function as a red blood cell, but it is still all there. What's more, with the right messaging it can still create any cell in the body. It is this process that was used to clone Dolly the sheep and this, my friends, is one reason why more primitive animals than us can regenerate limbs: they have stronger blood.

Becker went further. He messed around with electricity in salamanders and other animals and made them grow extra limbs and even heads. Using tiny electrodes he *re*-reversed the polarity at injured limbs and stopped them regenerating. Then he showed that higher animals, such as rats, can sometimes regenerate limbs, especially if he provided the injury site with an extra boost of electricity. He noticed that this power diminishes as the rat gets older and the injury gets more severe. As he worked with more evolved animals, he noticed that this regeneration reduced, along with the ability to generate a strong DC regenerative current and nucleated red cells.

Finally, he came to the conclusion that the more energy a species has spent on creating a big brain, the less ability it has to regenerate. Humans, with the largest brain per size of any large animal, have been left with the regenerative short straw.

Regeneration is a fact of life, but what is remarkable about people is the fact that we cannot do it in our limbs more readily. Regeneration is just embryology and the processes involved are the same. It is the same DNA, using the same pathways and the same messaging system. We regenerate every time we heal a cut or broken bones and, on a micro-level, we do this all the time in our body, a million times a day. Cells in our gut are constantly regenerating and forming a new gut lining, our bone marrow is constantly regenerating our blood and immune system, and our internal organs are certainly engaged in ongoing repair and replacement as cells wear out.

There are certain tissues that cannot regenerate, and the most devastatingly injurious of these are the brain and spinal cord. Injury here can result in a stroke or paralysis with no hope of regeneration – the cells are too specialised to wind back their embryological clock.

As I have said, the electricity that Becker showed in injured limbs wasn't the same as nerve impulses. It was constant, a DC current rather than the up-and-down AC current of nerves. Becker was unsure where it came from but a visiting doctor from the military wondered if it was the same mechanism as worked in Acupuncture – was this what the Chinese called Qi?

Part I

The Science of Acupuncture

or, What God Forgot
to Tell Surgeons

Genesis

In the beginning was a cell, a fusion of sperm and egg, Yang into Yin. Individually they were nothing, but combined they could conquer the world.

This was you, your cell… Maybe, deep inside you, it still exists?

The story of how that cell became you is the most amazing story ever told. It is a story that has not only created the astronomical complexity of our brains and the virility of our hearts, but is also responsible for civilisations and art, love won and life lost.

The cell contains everything within it to produce this, and yet it is invisible. How did it do this? You may think you know the answer in genetics, but you only have half the story.

The genes are like a great library, but a great library needs organisation. The story of this organisation is also the story of Acupuncture, explaining how the body creates and maintains order out of chaos. For the story of Acupuncture is the story of life itself, and it is only now, as modern medicine unravels the interactions between cells, that we understand what the ancient Chinese physicians knew: that the space between the cells is as important as the cells themselves.

The Single-Cell Universe

When your cell first starts it is in a world of space: a cellular being floating in the primordial soup of the fallopian tubes. It has just emerged from its own Big Bang: the moment of fusion of sperm and egg that has created your universe. It knows no up, no down, and it has no reference to right and left, back or front, for it has no need. As a single cell it is required only to survive in its dark space.

Soon it divides. Then these two cells divide again, and again, and again, until it is a ball of cells, a *morula* (Latin for the mulberry fruit it resembles), and an awareness is beginning within the cells that there is a spatial relationship with other cells. There is the embryogenesis of organisation. Within a few days the outer and inner cells of the morula start differentiating. They are performing individual roles. They are specialising.

The cells are responding to their relative positions by subtly altering their function. Those in the centre begin to secrete fluids. An egg is forming and the inside of this egg is even named the Yolk Sac. Those cells on the outside become stronger, tougher, more like skin.

The process continues at an astonishing rate. Within a week there are thousands of cells. Now the ball of cells is tumbling down the walls of the womb. It grabs a place to hold on and burrows into the endometrium – the surface of the womb. The ball of cells now has not only an inside and outside but also a left and right, up and down, near and far.

The parts on the outside start forming the placenta; the inside divides and creates the embryo. The cells decide that one end will become the head, the other the tail. The primitive spinal cord appears, and one end becomes bulbous, the primitive brain. Cells stream off from either side and form organs and muscles. Tissues fold over themselves, bend and rotate, move from one end to the other. It should be chaos, but instead it is poetry in motion.

The result is a perfectly formed mass of ten trillion cells. That's ten thousand, thousand, thousand, thousand cells!

Each cell knows not only where it is but also what it should be doing and which cell it should be next to. They have formed structures of immense complexity: an upside-down gossamer-leaved tree of a lung, a million nano-filtration units in the kidney, and a brain that can organise life into human civilisation – and they have done all of this from one invisible cell.

All of this is possible because of those 23 double-stranded spirals of DNA, and an epic level of organisation. When cells lose this organisation, then what happens is called disease.

The nastiest, the most feared and the most incurable of all diseases is cancer. Cancer is called cancer because it is the Latin word for, and acts like, a crab, spreading outwards with its malignant claws. This is the defining aspect of cancer: its uncontrolled spread. These are cells that no longer know their position and role in the body. They have lost their connection to the body. They are no longer part of it; they have become the enemy of the body.

To understand how our cells stay connected, and why when we lose this we develop cancer, we have to look at the most ignored tissue in the body: fascia.

'A Name but no Form'

NANJING, ISSUE 38, 1ST CENTURY AD

Cancer spreads through *fascia* (see Appendix 1) yet, despite this, fascia is the great ignored substance of Western medicine.

Wikipedia merits fascia (pronounced 'fa-sha') with a mere 18 lines; textbooks of medicine ignore it completely,[1, 2] and its only contribution to Western medicine is that it sometimes gets inflamed (fasciitis) and it sometimes throttles parts of the body (compartment syndrome).

Despite this, every good surgeon respects fascia. Every nerve, muscle, blood vessel, organ, bone and tendon is covered in it, and it tells a surgeon where things should be. Incredibly (as difficult as this may be for surgeons to believe), God didn't put fascia there for surgeons, it was put there to enable the body to know where things should be, and what they should be doing.

Surgeons make good use of this biological ordering, though. So long as they stay in the plane of the fascia they will cause little damage. Minimally invasive (keyhole) surgery exists thanks to this exact property. It exploits the fascial envelopes to create large internal spaces for performing operations, such as laparoscopies: it is possible to put a camera into the abdomen, have a look around your liver, your guts, your private parts (if you're a woman) and leave without causing more than mild discomfort. In fact, this is so easy that sometimes doctors do it just to have a look. (Doctors, like most intelligent people, are curious and nosey creatures and can almost always justify having a look around.) This is all possible because of fascia and the compartments it makes in the body.

Even the simplest operation will focus on finding the fascial planes and then working around them: Langer's lines of the skin tell surgeons how the collagen in the skin is arranged and surgeons then cut along these to minimise scarring.

Chinese medicine, however, respects fascia as much as, if not more than, any surgeon. It devotes not one, but two, organs to this most universal of tissues: the *Pericardium* and the *Triple Burner*. However, Western medicine disputes that these organs exist.

Chinese and Western medicine can seem contradictory and confusing at times (see Appendix 2) but at least they agree on the existence of all the organs...*with the exception of these two*. The pericardium is seen as an inert fibrous sac in Western medicine, hardly what would constitute an 'organ', and the Triple Burner exists neither as a physical organ nor even a concept. However, neither does it appear to exist as a physical organ in Chinese medicine! In the 2000-year-old medical classic the *NanJing* (*The Classic of Difficulties*), the Triple Burner is enigmatically called 'the organ with a name but no form'.

The *NanJing* was so named because it set out to clarify issues raised by an even *older* medical textbook – the *HuangDi NeiJing* (*The Yellow Emperor's Classic of Internal Medicine*). Ironic, then, that this statement still creates debate amongst acupuncturists, while it firmly refuses to ever be an issue amongst Western doctors. No Western doctors have ever discussed the *koan* that is 'What form does the Triple Burner take?' because (for them) the Triple Burner doesn't exist.

Acupuncturists may not agree on what the Triple Burner is, but they do agree on what it does in the body. It behaves somewhat like a compost heap. At the bottom is the fresh manure, in the middle is the soil and at the top are the flowers and carrots. This happy harmony is how it has to be. Dung beetles and colons may not mind living in excrement, but flowers and people do. So it is with the body. The middle section is where we take the goodness from what we eat, the bottom section contains the well-rotted manure, and the upper section (heart and lungs) is where our flowers bloom.

(This may sound somewhat poetic, but poetry often contains deep truths in artistic form and this description happens to be an accurate yet extremely concise summary of the body.)

The Triple Burner is also the key to understanding Acupuncture, since it is none other than the patterns created and modelled in the body by fascia. Fascia, a substance that has no form of its own, takes the form of that which it is covering. Fascia is the defining aspect of our body; it sculpts muscles in the arm, organs in the body, even the walnutty surface of our brains. It is truly an organ with no form of its own, yet it is everywhere.

An important note about the word 'fascia' here, because the term seems to confuse people. It's nothing to do the walnut interior of a freshly waxed red sports car, or even with Hitler's insane policies. Fascia is Latin for 'bands together', for that is what it does – it binds together tissues. Imagine vacuum-packed vegetables, or white goods…or even meat. Meat is vacuum-packed because it keeps all the juicy goodness in. The body vacuum packs everything in the same way but it uses fascia instead of plastic. Take any organ, muscle or body part and it will be vacuum-packed in fascia.

However, the vacuum in the body lies *between* the fascial layers. In health, the space between the layers is squashed together like an unopened supermarket plastic bag. We know the space exists to put our groceries in, but we have to open it first.

In our body the same is true; if you puncture a lung the fascial layers of lung and chest wall will naturally stay stuck together because the body maintains a negative pressure between the two. However, sometimes a 'valve' can form in the injured lung tissue that can stop air leaking back into the lung. As a result, the pressure between the fascial layers rises and the space opens up in the same way as your plastic bag at the supermarket checkout. Exactly the same principle is used by surgeons with keyhole surgery, but in the case of the punctured lung the condition is uncontrolled and dangerous. This condition is known as a *pneumothorax* and can actually kill people. The fascia itself is tiny, thin, almost transparent, but because it encases the lungs it has enormous power…the power to kill, but also, as we will find, the power of health.

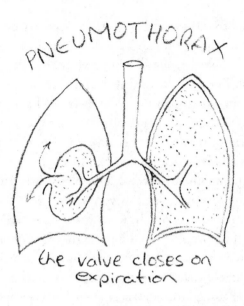

Fascia is a type of connective tissue, Western medicine's apt description of tissue that physically connects things. Connective tissue also includes bones, cartilage and even blood. Connective tissue has a matrix made and supported by the cells living within it. In bones, cartilage and fascia, this matrix is rich in collagen – a fact that is extremely important (blood is unusual in having a liquid matrix called *plasma*).

Fascia connects organs to muscle, to spine, to nerves... It surrounds bone and underpins skin. You find it in, around and on organs, sometimes in duplicate or even triplicate layers. Fascia is everywhere in the body and it is extremely strong. So strong that in the days of Björn Borg and John McEnroe, professional players' tennis strings were made from the fascia from the gut of a cow! Surgeons even use fascia from sheep's gut (although confusingly known as *catgut*) to tie surgical knots. Fascia is impenetrable to almost all biological substances, and not only is it an electrical conductor *and* resistor, but it also generates its own electricity: fascia is piezoelectric![3]

Fascia is so impermeable that almost everything slides down it: water, air, blood, pus and even electricity. It is this impenetrability that makes it so important and so useful to surgeons, for fascia creates compartments, unique areas in the body that act with a shared purpose.

The Triple Burners themselves are not so mysterious when fascia is considered. They are the compartments of the chest, abdomen and pelvis and the unique metabolism that occurs in each. (Technically they are the pleuropericardial, intraperitoneal and retroperitoneal compartments, but this is a bit of a mouthful.)

Between chest and abdomen sits the diaphragm, a thick layer of muscle surrounded on each side by a layer of fascia which isolates your heart and lungs from your abdomen. Between the kidneys, pelvis and abdomen sits another thick layer of fascia. What divides these areas is the same thing that divides all the parts of the body – fascia – but between these areas it is thicker. This fascia acts to lock in the metabolism of each area and, as a result, each of these areas starts to behave with a shared purpose.

These are the areas of the Three Metabolisms, what has been translated from ancient Chinese texts as the Triple Burner. The *NanJing* may have stated that it has no form, but that does not mean that it has no physical reality, and fascia is what creates it.

Fascia is not only the organ of the Triple Burner, or the key to surgeons performing their magic; it is also why Acupuncture works. As we shall see, fascia is absolutely vital to how the body forms – without it we would be an amorphous mess of jelly. Western medicine struggles with Acupuncturists' ideas of channels in the body, whilst inadvertently using the exact same system in their descriptions of anatomy and surgery. It is like a computer technician laughing at the absurd idea of electricity running invisibly in wires whilst replacing your hard-drive.

However, this oversight can be excused, for there is still no universal explanation within Western medicine for Acupuncture channel pathways. The meridians* of the body sometimes follow

---

* The original voyagers who returned with stories of Acupuncture from the East struggled to convey the meaning of the Chinese medicinal concept of 'Jing luo' – channels and collaterals. At the time, a well-meaning interpreter compared its interweaving network with the imaginary meridians of latitude and longitude, and the word 'meridian' stuck. It is a poor translation, however, and channel is a much better one, which is why I will refer to them as channels from now on.

nerves, but not always; many of them are found in the curves at the end of bones but then don't follow the bones themselves; they follow muscles and tendons most faithfully, but then play away from home when it suits them. There is definitely some relationship with what are called the 'fascial compartments' in the body, but this breaks down when the compartments end.

Countless bodies have been dissected, probed, dyed, irradiated and cooled by anatomists and they have found exactly…

Nothing.

This lack of objective existence of the meridians has been used as a powerful tool to dismiss their existence.

Western medicine may have missed the obvious, what has been under surgeons' fingers the whole time, their best friend, the one they can rely on in times of need, the map that guides their travels. When anatomists (and surgeons) looked for Acupuncture channels they ignored the one thing that was everywhere, covering everything, connecting everything, almost transparent and invisible, yet immensely strong: fascia. It was like a man looking for his glasses when they were on his face.

Fascia explains these Acupuncture channels perfectly. Furthermore, fascia explains the multitude of tinier pathways that Acupuncture theory teaches – what Acupuncturists call the *Jing* and the *luo*, the large channels and the tiny channels. Fascia explains why there are almost an infinite number of 'points', since fascia is everywhere. It explains how you can use the main fascial planes to predict where these main points will be, and how the channels will behave.

It goes further still. Fascia explains Qi, the ancient idea of a 'life force' that drives our existence. As we shall see, it explains it not in elusive and archaic terms but in hard science, science that now powers the most exciting medical avenue of the modern era – stem cell research. Fascia fleshes out Qi into morphogens, super-powerful substances in our body that guide us from cells into complex beings and are being shown to be central in cancer.

Most intriguingly, fascia explains the internal pathways, the pathways of Qi through the body that connect the internal organs before emerging on the outside through the channels on the arms and legs. These pathways, detailed for thousands of years in medical canons, appear to be almost random, but are critical in Acupuncture theory. They are the conduit by which Qi moves from the outside to the inside and why a point on the arm can affect the stomach or kidney. These paths become self-evident when you map the pathways of fascia.

Fascia is the overlooked link between Acupuncture and anatomy.

4

The Triple Helix

The principal ingredient of fascia is collagen. Collagen is found everywhere in the body. It forms not only our fascia, but also tendons, ligaments, the cartilage in our joints; it is present in artery walls, gives bones their tensile strength, and forms the connective tissue within the organs. It even allows you to see, forming the lens of the eye, and heal, forming scar tissue. It is no surprise then that collagen is the most abundant protein in our bodies, making up about a third of our total body protein.

Collagen fibres are not only the most common type of protein in the body, they also have remarkable properties.

Collagen is a triple helix. Most people are familiar with the double helix structure of DNA, so the triple helix of collagen requires just a little more imagination. This triple helix is formed from collagen sub-units, called tropo-collagen, which then spontaneously self-assemble. Three triple helix strands of collagen then spontaneously form another triple helix to create a 'super helix' which is called a microfibril. Finally, these fibrils are laid down along lines of stress.

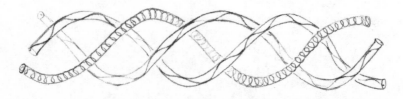

The whole array means that collagen is a semi-crystalline structure; that is, there is a regular repeating order of atoms in two dimensions.[1] This is important for the electrical properties of collagen.

Collagen is essential to the body, and the process of making collagen relies heavily on vitamin C. This is why sailors on long voyages used to bleed excessively from their gums: the wounds wouldn't heal because scar tissue is made from collagen, and their poor diet provided few vitamins. Captain James Cook realised the importance of fresh fruit, despite not knowing about vitamins, and would raid tropical islands for their bounties of fresh fruit. His sailors' new-found strength allowed him to circumnavigate the globe on the *Endeavour* and complete the type of journeys which have been immortalised in the adventures of Captain James Kirk and the *Enterprise*!

Collagen is not only the substance that glues the body together, it is also the substance that antiquity used to glue things together. *Colla-* comes from 'kolla', the Greek for 'glue', and *-gen* is short for 'genesis/creator'; and so collagen means 'glue creator'. In ancient times the skin and sinews of animals were boiled to down to make gelatine, which is pure collagen, to be used as glue.

The structure of collagen is created at an atomic level and this gives it enormous strength – per weight it is as strong as steel! This strength is vitally important since it is the base material in bones, arteries, muscles, tendons and fascia.

Collagen's strength is so great that it can become a problem. Fascia arranges the body into 'compartments', areas enclosed by fascia in which the only entry and exit points are narrow conduits for vessels and nerves. This serves an important role because it protects the contents within from spreading infection and also clearly delineates one part of the body from another. The compartments are analogous to rooms in a house where the only way in and out is through small windows or doors. Sometimes, injury can make the contents swell up. The strength of the collagen in the fascia will not yield to this rise in pressure and if there is no release then eventually it will cut off the blood supply. When this happens the contents become starved of oxygenated blood, swelling further as the cells start to die, in what becomes a vicious circle. The only treatment for this is a rather brutal procedure called fasciotomy, where the surgeon cuts open the fascia, releasing the pressure and allowing blood to get back in again.

Collagen not only has great tensile strength, it also has electrical properties that are all but ignored by Western science. Collagen has properties that include piezoelectricity, the ability to generate tiny electrical currents when an object is deformed. The sparks in cigarette lighters produce their magic by deforming tiny quartz crystals in the same process. That means that every time we move any part of our body we are creating tiny electrical currents.

The effect of weak collagen can be seen in the tragically beautiful blue eyes of babies with a disease called *osteogenesis imperfecta*. The whites of their eyes appear blue as the collagen is weak and allows light back through to reveal the colour of the underlying veins. The name of the disease, however, is Latin for 'imperfect bone creation' and usually presents itself with frequent broken bones in babies.

Bone has two types of strength: it is both hard and incompressible and also has great tensile strength. The former properties arise from the *hydroxyapatite* crystals, made of calcium and phosphate, which give bone its white sheen. Tensile strength is the ability to resist being broken and, surprisingly, it is not the crystals that create this but the collagen. The crystals are there to make the collagen 'stiff'.[2] When the bone is stressed the collagen keeps it strong and the hydroxyapatite crystals make it hard and inflexible.

The lines of stress in bone are normally well demarcated; when you land from a jump the pressure is transmitted along your skeleton in certain predictable ways. The body responds to these lines of stress logically by strengthening the bone in these directions. These lines are visible on X-rays as *trabeculae*, fine white lines in the bone which, when disturbed, are useful markers for spotting subtle fractures. Since collagen is not visible on an X-ray, the white lines are not collagen but are the chalky crystals of calcium and phosphate which have been laid down to add a marble-like hardness.

In fascia, muscles and tendons there are no crystals that are visible on an X-ray. In fact, these tissues are difficult to visualise with any imaging apart from ultrasound. However, the same process is occurring: the collagen fibres are laid down so that they are along stress-lines, giving it enormous tensile strength. Collagen in the form of cowgut is, after all, the substance with which Björn Borg won five Wimbledon Championships.

In bone, though, what collagen does is more remarkable than provide strength. Collagen is semi-crystalline and one of the properties of crystals is that they are piezoelectric. Bone is also piezoelectric and (as one author puts it): 'it has been shown that after decollagenation of bone no piezoelectric effect is observed. The major contributor to the piezoelectricity in bone is therefore the collagen.'[3]

The Spark of Life

Piezoelectricity is what allows your cigarette lighter to produce that tiny spark. It is static electricity created by bending a crystal, and it is being created all the time in our body.

The importance of the piezoelectric effect in the bone is still being elucidated. We know that it is the orientation of the collagen fibres that stimulates bone growth.[1, 2] The tiny electrical currents produced by this deformation of collagen stimulate the bone cells, called osteoblasts, to lay down more bone.[3] The way in which this occurs is, in theory, quite simple. When, for instance, you land from a jump the bones in your legs subtly bend and flex to absorb the shock. This flex is felt right the way through the bone, but the areas under most stress will flex the most. The collagen fibres in these areas will deform the most and so produce more electrical charge. This charge will then be detected by bone cells (osteoblasts), which will start laying down new crystals onto the collagen fibres. The result of this is that the bone in this area becomes harder and less flexible: the bone is stronger exactly where it needs to be.

This process is occurring all the time. Even subtly shifting your weight while reading this has caused this effect. The reason that astronauts lose so much bone mass when they go into space is because they lose this piezoelectricity. Without any gravitational stress on their bones the collagen stops producing any electricity. Even rigorous daily exercise cannot make up for the constant stressing produced by gravity. After a year in space astronauts are so fragile that the bones of these ultra-fit soldiers are like those of geriatrics. In space, astronauts lose *at least* 1 per cent of their bone per month[4] and nothing seems to be able to stop this.

This piezoelectric effect is what Dr Becker exploited to produce his bone-healing machines, and electricity and bone growth have become so linked within the scientific world that there are now hundreds of scientific papers on this. The UK's leading orthopaedic hospital in Stanmore routinely uses electrical devices to aid bone healing.[5]

The science of this is still poorly understood. However, what is definitely known is that collagen produces electricity, and electricity guides bone growth.

There is no reason to think that the collagen in the rest of the body isn't producing electricity when it is deformed. It is a property of collagen that produces the electricity, not of the bone, and the collagen elsewhere in fascia is exactly the same type. Collagen in fascia is laid down along lines of mechanical stress – every time it is stretched or moved it will generate tiny electrical charges. This electricity is completely ignored by Western medical doctors – ask any doctors about it and you will almost certainly be met with blank looks. Yet it is quite astonishing that the connective fabric of our body, the tissue that wraps and joins our entire body, is in effect an interconnected, living electrical web. This is so similar to the ancient Chinese descriptions of Acupuncture channels and Qi that it is remarkable.

Collagen is not only an electrical producer, it also has very interesting conduction properties: it is a semiconductor.[6] In other words, it behaves not quite like an insulator and not quite like a conductor. These are the same properties that give computers their 'intelligence'.

The structure of collagen suggests further properties that are on the edge of our current understanding of the body. Collagen is a triple helix and there is speculation (although no research) that it will conduct electricity much better down its length than across it. If this was the case then it would mean that the microstructure of fascia may have far more order and importance that we give it credit for.

The interesting electrical properties of collagen are intriguing, since everything in the body is electric. On the surface of every cell sits a pump that is as vital to life as your lungs are. The pump constantly throws out three sodium ions in exchange for letting two potassium ions in. This creates a net charge of negative ions within the cell, resulting in a tiny electrical charge across the cell. Without this charge the cell cannot function, and within minutes of this pump stopping working the electrical charge would disappear and the cell would swell up and die!

Electricity is essential to life.

The effect of electricity within the body moves beyond the grind of cellular existence. Nerves in the body use it to transmit information, muscle uses it to force contractions, and the brain uses it to think. The heart's rhythm comes from an electrical pacemaker, and the eyes even use electricity to register photons.

As Becker[7] would say, we really are 'Body Electrics', constantly emitting and absorbing an invisible silent energy that permeates all around us at the speed of light.

Every physiological process, every movement, every thought could be seen to have a twofold basis in reality: a physical reality and an energy reality. When the heart beats, the physical movement can be felt with your hand, or seen using ultrasound, but the electrical reality can be seen even more clearly with an electrocardiogram (ECG). Western medicine relies upon this test so often because in many ways this energy reality is more real than the physical reality, and is certainly easier to measure.

Increasingly, science is realising that electricity not only governs how we function, it also governs how we form. Electricity has been shown to tell stem cells where to move to, one of the most vital aspects of embryology.[8] The ability of electricity to mend broken bones is an expression of this, since bone healing is an example of regeneration and our ability to reform.

In the midst of this electrical world sits collagen, omnipresent and connecting to everything. It is accepted within Western medicine as the key constituent of our connective tissue, its strength supporting our body. As both an electrical semiconductor and an electrical generator of piezoelectricity, collagen's pre-eminence in the body may go beyond its mechanical strength. Instead, collagen should be seen as an electrical super-substance, a semiconducting, piezoelectric, bio-helix, holding, generating and even directing body electricity.

An electrical force held in a fabric into which our body is woven: this is science that is beginning to sound like Chinese medicine and Qi.

What is Qi?

No word has been so misunderstood in the West as Qi. This is partly a failure in translation, not only of the word but of culture and meaning too. The Chinese may have been intransigent, in the same manner in which they guarded the secrets of silk, but equally important has been a failure of the West to *try* to understand.

The word Qi is used in many forms apart from the medical sense and it is useful to look at how Qi is used elsewhere in the Chinese language. Written Chinese uses characters rather than letters and often combines characters to create different words. Each part of the new word is known as a *radical*. In the case of 'Qi', there are literally hundreds of words that have been formed using Qi as a radical.[1]

What all these words share is that 'Qi' is used in place of the English word 'air' or possibly 'space'.[1] For instance: '*qi*dianquang' means *air*boat (hovercraft), '*qi*beng' means *air* pump. In terms of etymology, Qi therefore appears to be a homologue for air...which makes you wonder why the ancients would have used a word such as Qi in relation to the rather solid thing that is the human body.

There is air in the human body, of course. There is air in the lungs and air dissolved into the blood and body fluids. This air is mainly in the form of oxygen and carbon dioxide, but there are trace amounts of nitrogen and other gases. Air in the form of carbon dioxide and oxygen is the fundamental basis of our metabolism – in fact these two gases alone can be used in scientific tests to elucidate our total body 'metabolism' over any given period.

Did the ancient Chinese have this in mind when they were talking about Qi?

The Chinese character for Qi also gives clues to its meaning. Many Chinese characters emerged from drawings, which over time became more simplified and lost some of their artistic credentials. Normally, however, they retain the essence of what was being conveyed. In the case of Qi, the character is written in two parts. The upper part represents steam, or air or possibly even clouds. The lower part is the character for rice which is being cooked; it is drawn as rice which is literally popping open.

Dr Jwing-Ming Yang, in his excellent DVD series entitled *Understanding Qigong*,[2] explained this character very succinctly. The ancient Chinese were merely drawing one of the simplest equations in medical science:

food + air = energy

glucose + oxygen = water + carbon dioxide + energy

$$C_6 H_{12} O_6 + 6O_2 = 6H_2O + 6CO_2 + Energy$$

The character of Qi represents this combining of the rice and air to create energy...which in a biological sense *is* Qi!

Which is correct? Is Qi metabolism, or is Qi 'air' or 'space'? The answer is that both are correct and more. Metabolic energy, in a sense, is defined by air; cut off the air supply to an organism and both its Qi and metabolism will disappear. However, Qi is too broad to be a substance; it is more a concept, which is one reason why Western science has struggled to pin it down. It shares more with philosophy than with science, with concepts or abstractions.

Abstractions remain the root of our scientific rationale, however. The simplest abstraction of all is into subjective and objective, the idea that there is a world outside of us which is somehow real and the world within us which is imaginary. This abstraction remains at the heart of the scientific principle because it posits that the outside reality can be tested and the results found to be reproducible. For instance, the principle of gravity appears to be always true in the outer world, but in our subjective world this is not always the case (for example, dreams are not always about real situations).

Qi is an abstraction that straddles these two worlds because Qi is the force created by the objective world that powers our subjective world. Qi is more than metabolism; Qi is intelligent and organised metabolism. It is the difference between *a* fire, and the fire in a jet engine: one just creates heat; the other creates heat that is channelled and focused. This difference is extremely important to understand: metabolism is dumb; Qi is intelligent.

As we shall see, Qi is more like the production from a large power station than a jet engine. A power station, a complex and large building, takes fuel and converts it into a very powerful yet subtle substance called electricity which runs in relatively thin wires. The energy is present throughout the process but gets increasingly concentrated to serve the purposes of the station. Qi in the body does this too and the concentration occurs not in wires but in channels in the body formed between fascia. If you looked at the power station without understanding about this invisible electrical force, you may come to the conclusion that the thin wires that left it were rather unimportant. You could make the same mistake with the body.

Qi as intelligent metabolism becomes a very large subject. The science of metabolism is immense, covering large swathes of biochemistry and physiology…but very little anatomy. What Acupuncture and fascial Qi theory promises is to combine these two, to allow form and function to follow each other. It is like a new branch of medicine, apart from the fact that it is not – we are just rediscovering the oldest medicine in existence.

To understand this better we need to go back to the beginning of time again, this time not in the dark spaces of the fallopian tubes but in one of the weirdest places on Earth – the laboratory at the Roslin Institute.

Cloning Sheep with Qi

When the scientists at the Roslin Institute in Edinburgh sparked Dolly the Cloned Sheep into life it was a truly stupendous achievement.

Cloning is not simple, regardless of how it looks in the pages of the *Daily Mail*. To create a cloned creature the scientists take an unfertilised egg from the mother. Since the DNA within this egg is only half complete, they remove it. Into this empty egg they then inject the DNA from one of the mother's cells. This DNA is complete, but they have a problem: it is also mature. As Dolly's 'mother' had grown, her DNA had matured too, and in the process lost the unbounded potential of youth.

The 'mother' DNA may have been programmed to be a skin cell on the hand, or a freckle, or a liver cell, but in the process of becoming mature it has turned on certain DNA and locked off most of the rest. In order for this DNA to produce a new Dolly the scientists have to unlock this DNA, winding back the clock to make it think it is young again. (This last point is important – wicked witches in fairy tales clamoured for this type of thing and, as we shall see, winding back the clock is not meant to be done; factals create massively different results from very similar starting positions – think DNA. Trying, but failing, to wind back the clock to get the exact starting position is why the bizarre aberrations in cloning happen.)

The ingredients of life may have all been put into place, but that did not mean that life was present. The cell consisted of a new egg cell with the mature maternal DNA unlocked within, but there was still no life, and this is where it gets weird…

Dr Frankenstein was right. He wildly overestimated how much electricity you would need but had exactly the right idea. The scientists at Roslin used a dose of electricity so small that it would barely disturb dust; it turned out there was no need for rickety lightning conductors perched atop gothic mansions. The tiny jolt of electricity did something truly astonishing: it kicked the cell into life!

I am sure the irony of using Dr Frankenstein's methods was not lost on the scientists who created Dolly, a sheep who was incidentally named in honour of Dolly Parton's twin assets. The process was not as smooth as is suggested: it took 277 attempts to make Dolly and in the process they created monsters of various proportions and shapes. Cloning causes truly freakish things to happen: giant creatures, dwarves, true mutants with multiple heads and too many limbs. Cloning is playing with the very building blocks of life and it is no wonder that it causes the delicate flower of organisation to go haywire.

Regardless of the ethical considerations, the implications of this are truly staggering: life can be created with electricity!

What is it about electricity that enables it to produce life? It is a question that moves to the very centre of our existence, for our lives are governed by electricity. The fingers typing on this keyboard are doing so by electrical charges moving down from my brain. My muscles are contracting as a result of electrical charges. These very thoughts are mirrored in electrical activity in my brain. Our life is electric, and what is bio-electricity if not concentrated metabolism, pure bio-energy, what Chinese medicine sees as Qi?

The parallels between Qi and electricity are intriguing. Science often balks at the idea of Qi as a vague invisible force but is quite happy to believe in the vague invisible force of electricity.

Vague? We all know that electricity travels in power lines, but when you place a fluorescent bulb near a power line it will glow. Is the electricity in the air or the line? If it is in the air then how is it travelling? If it's electrons then where do they end, and if it's a force field why do they talk about electrons?

Electricity constantly poses more questions than it answers.

Invisible? Similarly, the argument that Qi cannot exist because we cannot see it is fallacious. Qi is visible in the same way that electricity is visible: through its effects. Anyone claiming that pixie dust is moving an electric motor would be laughed at, since we all know the truth. But! It is not the electricity you see, only the *effect* of the electricity. It is the same in the body: all your actions, whether it be sleeping, laughing or running, are an effect of Qi. That is the proof.

'Fine!' you may say. 'What about lightning? You can see that!'

The same is true of metabolic energy or Qi, though. Humans emit light; it is just so faint that only machines can measure it. Strangely, it appears to come most strongly out of the fingernails in a similar way to which 'evil-Qi' is seen in popular fiction (such as *Star Wars*' evil Emperor).

The light emitted is called *biophotons* and it is an accepted scientific fact.[1-5] All living creatures emit this light, and whilst some creatures emit visible light too, the mechanism involved appears to be different. Eerily, again just like *Star Wars*' Emperor, these biophotons are in the same spectrum of light as the light from lightning: the near-ultraviolet part of the spectrum. Fritz-Albert Popp, a German scientist, believes that these biophotons are an expression of Qi, and represent an ability of the cells of the organism to stay together.[2]

The parallels with Qi are definitely there. The channels of Qi in the body end at the fingernails and toes, the same places where biophoton emission is strongest. When people get sick or old the rate of biophotons has been found to increase,[3] and the same happens on the same side of the body as a stroke. Acupuncture has been shown to balance this out in stroke patients.[4] Paradoxically, it appears that the more biophotons that are released, the less health, or Qi, the organism appears to have: it is almost as though they are losing their Qi.

It is not known whether biophotons are Qi, but what is definitely known is that most of them emerge from the DNA of our mitochondria, the powerhouses of our cells and the origin of energy in our body. Some researchers think they are an indicator of free radical damage but, then again, we don't really know. Some studies also show that biophotons are *coherent*.[5] Coherence is a quantum term to explain how energy seems to communicate with itself, light that is in sync with itself. Light having intelligence or memory may appear to be of interest only to quantum physicists, but in the body this is incredible!

The research into this is so poor that we are still really in the dark. The problem is that to measure biophotons you have to measure light at one-thousandth the intensity of what a person can see. This means that you need very expensive equipment and people who are willing to do an awful lot of sitting around.

Biophotons may be a physical manifestation of Qi, or they may just be a by-product of cellular reactions. Further research is needed and until then biophotons remain more of a curiosity than any evidence of Qi. What they do show, though, is that, like electricity, our bodies can produce light and that this light is altered in disease states.

The argument against Qi existing therefore becomes an argument born of stubbornness. If Qi is invisible it is only because energy generally is. If Qi is vague and difficult to pin down it is again no different to electricity. To argue against the existence of Qi is to argue against life itself. What powers life?

Qi.

Western medicine concerns itself with the minutiae of the cells, the way in which oxygen and sugar combine in the mitochondria to produce ATP, the incredible machinery that powers each cell, the cells that group together to form organs, muscles, bones, testes and even the drums in our ears. Only in embryology does it concern itself with the question 'How?'

How do all the cells work together? What drives them to cooperate? Embryology goes into more and more detail about growth factors and messengers and cell types until the description is a complicated mess. Qi is much more useful as a concept because it is unifying. Instead of Chinese medicine concerning itself with minutiae, it concentrates on the *innate ability* of our cells to work together and function cooperatively. To create teamwork that is more than the individual. To bind together to produce you, warts and all.

Qi is the energy produced by each cell, the binding force between those cells and the work they produce: the sum of all metabolism. For want of a better phrase, the term *life force* comes to mind. There is no comparable force within Western medicine. Many people try to equate Qi with nerve and brain energy, but nerves cannot explain organogenesis, the process by which organs create themselves and then work harmoniously, and why incredible organisation has formed in the embryo way before any nerves have appeared (in the fourth week).

Qi is more than merely cellular metabolic energy; it is developmental energy, cooperative energy.

If a football team analogy was used, then Qi would be both the energy of each player *and* the invisible bonds that bind the team together. These bonds may be sounds (i.e. words and commands), meaningful glances, understandings, or even that certain *je ne sais quoi* that brilliant teams have; but what these bonds have in common is that they are ephemeral and mainly invisible. Football teams train for hours, days, months, years…even decades to build up this rapport, yet if you asked the manager to show this 'Team Qi' then he would shrug his shoulders and tell you to watch them play.

Yet without this energy the team is impotent. You could place the 11 greatest players of all time on a pitch, and without the invisible energy of team-ship they could be beaten by a well-organised pub team. The same is true a trillion times over for the greatest team of all, the 11 trillion cells that make up 'Team You'.

This is why Qi is so important, because it is unifying rather than reductionist. There is no equivalent concept within Western medicine and this is one reason why it opens up avenues of healing that do not exist in the West.

If Qi is intelligent metabolism – team metabolism – then what would Qi consist of in Western science? Which forces in the body would create it? It would have to be a product of cellular energy, organ energy, and then, most importantly for Acupuncture, the energy of communication and of intelligent cooperation.

The Perfect Factory

The metabolism and energy production of cells has been well studied by Western medicine. In fact, the physiology of energy production is known to the atomic level and it is truly incredible.

The reality is that each of us at a cellular level consists of not one but two creatures. Each animal cell consists of the *eukaryotic* cell within which lives *mitochondria*. These two organisms fused billions of years ago and this fusion resulted in an explosion of evolution. The mitochondria, however, still maintain their own DNA and cell wall – some scientists even believe that they have sex.[1]

Every cell in your body has these little mitochondria in them. It really is the original beautiful relationship, over three billion years old and still going strong. Eukaryote and mitochondria are wholly dependent on each other to survive – a symbiotic relationship. The cells provide the mitochondria with everything they need: sugar, oxygen, a few amino acids and a cosy safe place to do what they do best. They nurture the mitochondria like precious children. In return the mitochondria take in sugar and oxygen and churn out molecules of adenosine triphosphate (ATP), cellular dynamite.

ATP powers just about every cellular action from muscle contraction, to nerve impulses, through heartbeats and on to ion pumps. ATP is the most important form of cellular energy but there are other molecules that the mitochondria produce. Without the mitochondria the cell is doomed; if cyanide poisons the mitochondria, death occurs in minutes.

The role of mitochondria goes beyond energy production, though. They are also instrumental in programmed cell death – apoptosis. Programmed cell death is one of the most important functions of the body. It literally stamps out your body in 3D: your fingers are formed because the cells in between them are told to die.

The mitochondria kill the cell by flooding it with calcium, and are told to do this either because the cell is old and defective, or because the cell is not part of the bigger plan of the body.

It is not surprising then that mitochondria themselves are implicated in cancer.[2] Failure to turn on this self-destruct mechanism will mean that the cells don't die when they are supposed to.

Early on in evolution the bizarreness of cell suicide (apoptosis) emerged at a time when cells started living together, and this moment in evolution coincided with mitochondria fusing with animal cells. Mitochondria allowed cells to live when grouped together, and for some reason at this point the mitochondria became not just the providers of life but also the bringers of death.*

However, the most important role for the mitochondria in adult life remains as the power stations of the cells. Mitochondrial defects are associated with lethargy, chronic tiredness, organ failure and early death. Mitochondria produce the energy that we use, but this isn't where our energy ends but rather where the energy *begins*.

The cell is much more than the power station. The cell has an immense database called DNA, housed in a nucleus. The DNA is read and then churns out messengers called RNA. These messengers then leave the nucleus to make proteins, and then these proteins spontaneously self-assemble to make the cell.

The beauty of this cannot be understated. Imagine a factory with a control centre that churns out instructions on how to build the parts of the factory: the bricks, pipes, cabling, roof, conveyor belts, nuts, bolts…the lot. Another part of the factory takes these messages and assembles these parts from bits hanging around. These bits then self-organise and go exactly where they are needed. The roof goes to the roof, cabling goes to where it is needed, and so on. The parts all join up in just the right way to keep the factory

---

*   For more on these quite magnificent organisms please read *Power, Sex, Suicide: Mitochondria and the Meaning of Life*.[3]

running perfectly and then even to make another factory which can do exactly the same thing. The factory takes everything it needs from around itself, not only producing very little waste but in the process producing many useful things. Then put several trillion of these perfect micro-factories together and turn them into a body!

The intelligence in this is immense. In nature, life is not the only self-forming substance: crystals too exhibit this same property. (Interestingly, the collagen network that binds us together within fascia has been compared with a liquid crystal mesh[4] that may go some way to explaining our ability to self-form.)

The cell then not only creates energy for itself, through enabling mitochondria, but also produces substances that enable the cell to work. Furthermore, it produces useful substances for the body to function as a whole, to be more than its parts. The cell's work is directed and intelligent. Just as the cell is self-forming, so multiple cells then group together in a common purpose to perform a shared role. When this purpose is vital, we call this an organ.

9

Organ Qi

The classic description of the division of labour of the body within both Chinese and Western medicine is into organs. One defining aspect of an organ is that it is surrounded by its own fascia, be it the pericardium around the heart, Gerota's fascia around the kidney or periosteum around the bone. This fascia both defines the organs and limits them. It encapsulates them but also constrains them. The cells within these fascial envelopes, forming these organs, all contain a common shared purpose which unites them – the functions of the organ.

This shared purpose has its own energy. In the heart it serves to move blood; the kidney energy is there to filter and remove waste products from the watery part of the blood; the lungs extract goodness from the air, and so on. Every cell in the organ works towards this shared aim, even though there are many different cell types.

For instance:

- in the heart, pacemaker cells create the first spark of electricity that starts the heartbeat

- then the conducting tissue cells transmit this spark

- the cells in a tiny region of the heart called the AV node slow this down to allow the atria of the heart to empty first

- then the pulse spreads out to the muscle cells of the ventricles which contract pushing blood out

- the cells that made the *chordae tympani* (the heart strings) pull to close the valves

- finally, the aortic valve opens and the blood rushes out.

This process occurs every second of every day. There are many different cells, with many different functions, but their unity of purpose creates a common energy. They have to work together as one, otherwise disease would erupt. If the pacemaker cells do not fire then the heart will not start, and will go too slowly or not at all.* When the conducting system cells get diseased then the heart misfires: if the muscle is damaged then the engine is weak, and if the valves go, then, just like your car, you get engine blowout.

All of these cells perform different roles – they have different parts of their DNA and different proteins working in them, they have had a different evolution, but, despite this, they work together in perfect harmony. They do this for a purpose.

This purpose is greater than the sum of its parts and we call it the *function of the organ*. It is a distinct entity that creates harmonic resonance, and this resonance can be measured by us or with machines. In the case of the heart, the electrical harmonies within this are easily read using an ECG, the mechanical harmony by feeling the pulse, and the harmony of the fluttering of the valves can be seen by using an echocardiogram.

The brain creates electrical waves that correspond to our state of consciousness. When the harmonic oscillation is at 3 Hz we feel sleepy, at 8 Hz we are either dreaming or awake, and at 30 Hz we are multitasking! The lung vibrates with every breath and can be measured with spirometry. A wave of contraction moves down the guts at a resonance of around 7 Hz. The kidneys produce their magic at such a nano-scale that no machine can measure the function of the nephrons, but these nephrons pulse with every beat of the heart.

The functions of the organs are so distinct that organs are able to be transplanted – they are interchangeable. When this is done, surgeons use the fascia to tell them where the organ ends.

The importance of this is that the organ has its own metabolism, its own energy: its own Qi. It is more than the sum

---

* Other cells can take over the pacemaker function but they pace more slowly.

of the individual cells' energy: it contains an organisational energy and it creates a much greater energy.

Chinese medicine also believes in this unity of purpose of organs but it measures the Qi of the organ instead of these other parameters. Qi is shown through the strength of a heart beating, or the ability of the lungs to take a deep breath, or the bladder to pee strongly, but it is also something more than these abstracted functions. Qi is the *totality* of the function of the organ. The Qi is the strength of the organisational energy in the organ, and those component parts: pulse strength, lung capacity, urine output – an aspect of this rather than this.

This organisation of the cells is called *physiology*, but when it goes wrong it becomes *pathology*. In the body, pathology and *disorder* are really the same thing, and disorder can be characterised in certain ways. Disorder of organisational energy can be weak and ineffectual, or too strong and invading; it can be going the wrong way, not going at all or just going plain crazy. However, these are not just the descriptions of how organisations can misbehave but also the descriptions that Chinese medicine gives to Qi pathology. When Chinese physicians talk about Qi pathologies, they could equally be talking about how organisation goes wrong in the body.

If the Qi (organisational energy) in the heart is too weak then it starts to beat weakly or slowly; if the Qi is too strong and it beats too powerfully then hypertension emerges and it *invades* and damages other organs such as the brain or kidney; if the Qi goes the wrong way you get arrhythmias which cause the heart to beat irregularly; crazy Qi gives you more serious arrhythmias and no Qi at all means you need to make your peace with God...

You can apply this to any organ, but each organ has its own dynamic resonance, its own organisation, and so the Qi within it is different. The Heart is Yang and full of electricity, but the Liver is Yin and full of blood (see Part III) so organisational energy problems here present differently and through the Qi of the blood.

In the Liver, if the Qi is weak then the Liver itself gets sludgy and fibrosed, causing the blood to stagnate (portal hypertension and atherosclerosis); if it becomes too strong it can affect the Liver's production of clotting factors which regulate how the blood moves in the body (too 'fast' and you get bleeding, too 'slow' and you get blood clots); it is also implicated in blood going 'crazy' (a condition known as disseminated intravascular coagulation (DIC) where the blood moves too 'fast' and too 'slow' at the same time).[1]

The Kidney relates to water and so the pathology of this organ is reflected in the fluid status in the body: weak Kidney Qi causes water to go backwards or overflow and you get oedema or fluid on the lungs; if the Kidney energy gets too strong its Qi can 'invade' and give you high blood pressure; and in some adrenal gland disturbances (for very good anatomical and endocrinological reasons, the adrenal gland is considered part of the Chinese Kidney) you get Qi behaving 'crazily'.

The Lungs manage our breath and so when its Qi goes the wrong way it causes us to cough; weak Lung Qi leads to breathlessness; and, rarely, the Lung Qi can get too strong and can 'invade' the heart.

A strong Gut gives us a strong digestion, so when its Qi is weak so is our digestion. When it rebels and goes the wrong way so does your food; when it is too strong and 'invades' it causes a build-up of Phlegm (what most in the West call fat).

The disorders of organisational energy in our body are further subdivided into what the ancient Chinese Taoists would have called the *10,000 things*: these are the countless diseases of Western medicine. This complexity can be incredibly powerful, allowing very specific treatments.

However, simplicity also has its own innate power. Qi, the organisational force of the body, moves according to simple laws, yet like water it carries with it different properties depending on its location. Water in rivers, oceans, lakes, streams, glaciers and even clouds remains water but has very different characters. Lakes are still, clouds rise, oceans roll, rivers flow. Despite these characteristics, water moves in predictable and simple ways. Qi behaves like this – it has different characters depending on where it is found but remains in essence the same thing. This simplicity allows very simple treatments based on its disorder. The basis of

Acupuncture relies upon this uniformity of Qi whilst celebrating its different manifestations.

Organ Qi in Chinese medicine does a lot more than simply provide a physical basis for the body; it also provides an emotional platform for the mind and body to interact. For instance, the Kidney in Chinese medicine handles our relationship with fear. It enables us to engage with fear appropriately. Escaped lions down the high street should cause our adrenals (part of the Kidney, in Chinese medicine) to go into overdrive but reading a book on lions shouldn't.

You may perceive and cognate the emotion of fear in the head, but it is the adrenal gland that enables this communication with the body. That record-breaking 100 metres away from the lion (real or imagined) is not produced by thinking fear, it is produced by *feeling* fear. Your body physically feels the adrenaline your adrenals release. The adrenaline has caused extra power in your muscles from an influx of calcium, sugar to be released from fat, and blood to be diverted from your gut to your vital organs. None of this happens 'in your head' – it happens in your body. Thinking 'fear' won't make this happen; you need adrenaline to create your mind–body interaction.

All the organs have strong emotional ties via hormones. The adrenals produce adrenaline; the gut, serotonin (a calming happy hormone); the liver cleans up histamine, the hormone of irritability; and the heart is affected by all the other hormones. You cannot feel fear to the same extent without your adrenals; when your liver fails you become irritable and twitchy (encephalopathic); and it is difficult to feel happy, content, replete when your gut is malfunctioning.

Each organ then has its own organising energy, its own Qi, but the Qi of these organs needs to inter-relate. A failing heart will cause the kidney to react by producing more stress hormones, a process that can cause the heart to fail further (the common class of drugs known as angiotensin converting enzyme (ACE) inhibitors work by interrupting this destructive feedback loop). A liver that that does not produce enough alpha-1 antitrypsin will cause destruction of the delicate lung tissue and lead to emphysema. Emphysematous lungs that fail to absorb enough oxygen will starve the heart of energy and cause it to weaken, which will cause the kidneys to stress, and so on… Everything is connected and the connections are equally as important as the organs.

One way in which the organs stay connected is through hormones released into the blood, but this plays little role in embryological development. Instead, there is another, more important, more primal force, which we look at in the next chapter.

10

How Qi Folds the Body

In the very early embryogenesis of the organism, communication was achieved by cell-to-cell contact. As the embryo developed and the cells began to number in their tens of millions, superhighways of information were needed. The fascial planes emerged from the middle embryological layer, the mesoderm, as a way of both delineating tissues and organs and enabling them to stay connected. After all, they were not given the name 'connective tissue' for nothing.

The publisher asked me to draw these fascial planes. I explained that it was like trying to draw clingfilm – you can only see what is underneath.

At first the fascial planes were simple but they rapidly became like origami. Origami starts simply but ends up fiendishly complicated. The starting point is a piece of paper with a single plane of existence – up and down. Simply by folding this plane, swans, elephants, airplanes and even paper people can be made.

Origami is about a single plane of existence and a lot of folding. The body has a middle layer that creates yet more complexity, but the principles of origami still hold – it must stay connected.

These connections persist in adult life as three simple layers (in three dimensions):

- the outer part, which forms skin and nervous system

- the inner part (the Yolk Sac), which forms gut and glands; and

- the middle part, which forms all else – blood, bone, fascia and muscle.

These three layers are named in Greek and are known, respectively, as ectoderm, endoderm and mesoderm.

The devil is, however, in the detail. Whilst in essence the body is simple, and this simplicity can still be seen in our primitive evolutionary ancestors, the sophistication of our bodies requires epic levels of folding. The gut folds over and over so it can squeeze 30 feet of tubing into our belly, the brain folds into itself to maximise the surface area it can use to process information, and the heart folds to accommodate the turbulent flow of blood. Every part of our body has been folded in some way.

Organs can thus appear very complex but all start from these same three layers, and their fascial planes are normally very simple. The lung grows out as a bud from your gullet and despite how complex the organ becomes its fascial connection remains this simple. The heart is nothing more than a convoluted tube, so its origini remains a tube. The kidney is more complex, consisting of two primitive precursor kidneys that fuse together – one end is plumbing and the other is the filtration unit. Furthermore, it has a large blood supply which brings its own fascia…the body may be origami but it isn't *that* simple!

The fascia defines and encapsulates organs, and we know that it is difficult for biological things to pass across fascia but relatively easy to pass along it. This is true of fluid, hormones, blood, air, even electricity. We know this because surgeons know and use this fact every day. Cancer's malignancy is defined by its perversion of this rule: in health, things travel *between* fascia not *through* it.

The organs are within the fascia, but they also connect with other organs. How do they know when to stop growing? Why do they not invade each other or steal their blood? The organs must communicate, not only to be able to grow together but also to live together. All that folding may be simple in essence, but *what* is telling the body to fold?

We know that organs secrete substances that affect other cells – our bodies are a seething mass of hormones constantly communicating messages to other cells and organs. Not only do glands such as the adrenal and pancreas produce hormones such as adrenaline and insulin, but our immune cells are constantly producing neurotransmitters, our heart cells diuretics, our gut serotonin, and so on. These hormones are transmitted in the blood and enable organs to communicate with the rest of the body simultaneously.

This form of communication is different to developmental communication that embryological theory envisages. Hormones travel to distant sites to exert their effects and need to do this quickly. Insulin produced by the pancreas goes to every cell in the body, and its transmission through the blood is necessary for its immediacy of effect. There would be little point in it slowly diffusing out from the pancreas because by the time this had happened the damage from high sugar levels would have been done. Furthermore, hormones by their nature exert their action at distant sites; their blood-borne nature means they have no specificity. The guiding forces of embryogenesis need to act locally, otherwise they risk causing anarchy.

Not only that, but whatever is guiding embryogenesis cannot be occurring entirely within the blood simply because early development of the embryo occurs before blood vessels are formed. In just the same way that primitive animals are bloodless, so are our embryological beginnings. Blood is only widespread in the embryo at the end of the fourth week, by which time there are at least 20,000 cells living in perfect harmony.

Inter-organ Qi, inter-organ developmental communication, must be another form of communication that is more primal and simple than hormones and predates nerves, a form that strangely enough involves Sonic Hedgehog, about which more later.

11

Tricky Dicky and Little Pricks

There are many problems with most theories of Acupuncture proposed by the Western scientific community. The primary problem always seems to emerge as a result of a failure to accept what the Chinese have to say about Acupuncture. One of the most commonly cited theories amongst doctors is the endorphin theory of Acupuncture. This was based on research that was done in the 1970s after the world was astounded by what Richard Nixon saw on his state visit to China. The Chinese, it appeared, were doing open-heart surgery with Acupuncture as anaesthesia!

It is worth pointing out that these operations were rarely done with Acupuncture anaesthesia alone. Rather, they were done with a combination of sedation and Acupuncture. The combination of these two allowed the operation to be done without a general anaesthetic and so was cheaper, still an important consideration in China. While it can be done manually, Acupuncture anaesthesia is done using electro-Acupuncture as otherwise somebody has to spend the entire time rotating the needle to stimulate the channel. The Chinese consider that the Acupuncture channel is being jammed, unable to function properly and so unable to transmit the pain/Qi.

Regardless of how Acupuncture anaesthesia works, the result of this was that Acupuncture was catapulted into the Western consciousness. Suddenly, the scientific community needed to provide answers about how placing a few needles into somebody's arm could allow you to do open-heart surgery. Western science being what it was, little attention was paid to what the Chinese taught, and Chinese is a difficult language to learn. (On a visit to China I struggled to understand how my attempts to ask for 'cha' could be mistaken for anything but tea. A friend put me right and explained that it has 24 different meanings depending on the tone used to pronounce it and the context. Apparently I could have been asking for a raft, a temple or simply been 'stuck'…)

The oral form of the language may be difficult, but the written form is practically impenetrable without years of study. Even the native Chinese argue about the meanings of characters and struggle to read the ancient texts.

What further hampered understanding was the way in which Acupuncture had been taught. Traditionally the knowledge was passed down through lineages: it was more of an oral than a written tradition. Practitioners often jealously guarded their 'secrets', fearing that that they would be stolen and their own practice would become obsolete.

In the 1960s Mao put an end to this. He forced the leading acupuncturists and herbalists to come together to form a corpus of medicine, what was to become known as Traditional Chinese Medicine. For this reason it is, ironically, not as traditional as it appears. Mao was both Communist and dogmatic, and this philosophy permeated through the whole of 1960s China. Chinese medicine was no different: spirit had no place in a world where people were seen as worker bees in a hive, and it was almost entirely purged from Chinese medicine. The great teachings of Chinese medicine placed spirit at the centre of our existence; Mao's Traditional Chinese Medicine saw spirit as decadence of the bourgeoisie.

The other great travesty that Traditional Chinese Medicine committed against the tradition of Chinese medicine was placing herbalism and Acupuncture within the same frame. The result of this was that Acupuncture became relegated to a subdivision of herbalism rather than a healing tradition in its own right. Concepts that worked in herbalism were transferred, such as warming the body or cooling the body, that had little prior use in Acupuncture.

Diagnosis was with tongue and pulses, but ignored the channels completely.

All these factors combined to create a situation in which the essence of Acupuncture had been both assimilated and destroyed in the same process. Maybe because of this, or maybe in spite of it, little knowledge was transferred to the Western scientists and doctors. It is not surprising then that despite determined investigation no evidence of Acupuncture channels was found. Western science gave its pronouncement on the issue: there were no channels; the primitive Chinese were deluded.

If only the scientists had immersed themselves in a little of Chinese philosophy they may have stumbled across one of the pearls of the classic Taoist scriptures:

A cup is only useful because of its emptiness.

So it is with the body. It is the space between cells, between organs and between fascia, where the Acupuncture channels lie. You cannot see them because they appear closed but they are still there. A channel, by definition, has the ability to be empty. In the body the Acupuncture channels appear empty because what they transmit is so powerful that you only need tiny amounts, whether that is growth factors (morphogens) or even electricity.

The blank that anatomical research had drawn in trying to identify the channels was precisely because they were looking for something, when what was to be found was next-to-nothing. It was the *space* within the body that allowed movement and growth. Drawing this blank on the channels, research moved swiftly on to what *was* there, and before long it was found that Acupuncture releases natural endorphins.

Endorphins are the body's natural painkillers. That high feeling you get from extreme exercise is caused by endorphins; it also causes the vomiting. Opium, morphine, diamorphine (heroin) and the like all work on the same receptors as endorphins, and they are fantastically good drugs. Effectively, almost all of Western medicine's best painkillers work on endorphin receptors. Research into Acupuncture had found that blood levels of endorphins increased when Acupuncture was given.

Western science had triumphed, the mystery was solved and everyone was advised that there was no magic to Acupuncture – it was just performing like a morphine injection, albeit a very curious one.

But! There were a few problems with this explanation. The main problem with the endorphin theory of Acupuncture is that it only predicted one effect, that of pain relief. The physiological effects of Acupuncture have been studied and vary from blood pressure lowering,[1] to heart rhythm regulation,[2,3] and on to airway opening.[4] Whilst these effects could be caused by endorphin release, their variety suggests effects through other mediators. In the case of the best studied and one of the most well-known uses of Acupuncture, in nausea,[5,6] there is no known effect from endorphins that could cause this. In fact, the opposite is almost certainly true: that opiates and endorphins produce nausea.

What the scientists proposed was a classic example of wrong thinking. A causing B does not mean B is how A works. My car engine creates a lot of heat, but it is not the heat *per se* that makes it work. Standing over my car and heating it is not going to get the engine moving.

In the same way, Acupuncture can release endorphins and these probably modulate some effects, but that does not mean that endorphins are how Acupuncture works. Giving endorphins won't work like Acupuncture.

The second problem with this theory is that endorphin release would have to be fairly massive to allow open-heart surgery. If performing open-heart surgery without a general anaesthetic was just a question of releasing some natural opiates then doctors could give a big injection of morphine and be done with it. Whilst this can be done (it is called 'general anaesthesia') it also causes the patient to go into a coma and stop breathing!

The Acupuncture and endorphin theory was never really accepted, but it was never really discarded either. Rather, it was merged with another theory that scientists offered. Again, this was a theory that revolved around explaining Acupuncture's effects away with something that Western science felt it understood and existed, and again it struggled in practical reality. It is called the 'gate-control' theory of Acupuncture.

The 'gate-control' theory of Acupuncture is a modification of the 'gate-control' theory of pain. The latter is actually quite a neat theory that explains why rubbing yourself after an injury seems to make it better. The 'gate' in 'gate-control' theory is located in the spinal cord. The spinal cord collects all the nerves from the body and it controls which signals will go up towards the brain, acting like a filter. For example, when you have been standing in the same place for a while you consciously forget the sensation from your feet – it is no longer important what you are standing on and so the nervous system eliminates this from your attention.

The nervous system does this in the spinal cord and also an area in the brain called the thalamus. The thalamus is like the secretary you find after you've got through the gate, up the path (spinal cord) and into reception (brainstem). Whether the message gets to see the boss in the cerebral cortex is now up to this secretary. Interestingly, the reason why smells can be so evocative is that smell is the only sense that bypasses the secretary (thalamus) and has direct access to the boss – your consciousness. Next time you notice the smell of freshly mown grass bringing back memories of childhood, it is because it has sneaked past the secretary and gone straight to your memory banks.

As you can see, the nervous system is quite complicated, but the 'gate' in the spinal cord is the place where the nervous system makes a decision about what goes up and what doesn't. Constant stimulation – 'feet are standing on something soft' – will eventually close the gate; whereas no stimulation – 'my feet are dangling in the air' – will leave the gate open to allow your brain to register when something gets added. This, the theory states, is why rubbing your arm after you've banged it helps the pain: the extra stimulation from the rubbing closes the gate.

As a theory of pain, this explains a little of why pain can be so variable, but it still fails to explain a lot of pain problems. As a theory of Acupuncture, it is desperate! Whilst it may explain some local pain relief effects, it cannot explain distal effects. It has no explanation as to why Acupuncture's effects persist for more than a few minutes, let alone months. Finally, it offers nothing to explain Acupuncture's other effects (anti-hypertensive,[1] anti-arrhythmic,[2,3] bronchial relaxation,[4] anti-emetic,[5,6] etc.), which are not related to pain.

The fact that this theory was accepted in any way by the medical establishment appeared to show the impossibility of ever reconciling Eastern and Western medicine. The problem was that there was no theory of how Acupuncture could work that fitted within the established medical-scientific view of the body, whilst being true to the Chinese concepts of Qi and channels.

Despite this, Acupuncture flourished and grew. It moved from hippy alternative to mainstream in just a few decades, and it did so competing with a free system (in the UK). It became so popular that it was co-opted by Western medicine, where it was stripped of its more 'esoteric' dimensions. The Chinese, however, remained unmoved. We were missing the obvious, they still insisted.

Whilst many doctors dismissed these Oriental concerns, research continued into what could possibly account for such a wildly different view of the body. Then, in 2001, a Dr Charles Shang of the Harvard Medical School published a paper that explained not only all of Acupuncture's effects but also what the Acupuncture points were.[7] It was a truly beautiful theory, building on lots of work by other researchers, taking what we know about the body through anatomy, physiology and embryology, listening to the Chinese, and then combining the two in a true moment of inspiration. He called his theory the Growth Control Theory of Acupuncture.

12

Human Fractals

The Growth Control Theory of Acupuncture is a bit of a mouthful but, in essence, it's what this book is about. Dr Shang drew from observations about Acupuncture points' positions and their functions to explain why they are where they are and do what they do.

The early part of the theory concerns embryology. In order to grow, the embryo needs organisation more than any other feature. The level of organisation required to make a human baby is quite simply staggering. In nine months a single cell will multiply until it is 10,000,000,000,000 cells. This alone is quite a feat, but while it does this it will organise itself into everything that we take for granted in good health.

There is some simple mathematics involved in organisation. To organise two people you need one line of communication; to organise three you need 1+2; to organise four you need 1+2+3; for 5 you need 1+2+3+4 and so on. By the time you get to 1,000,000,000,000 you will need 1+2+3+4...+ 999,999,999,999!

These are triangular numbers. They stack up like triangles:

I

II

III

IIII

As the number of people (or cells) increases it approaches n squared, where n is the number of cells. In the case of 1,000,000,000,000 cells this means there are approaching 1,000,000,000,000, 000,000,000,000 (1 septillion) lines of communication.

50

It's a ridiculously large number and quite clearly impossible to manage. The body, though, is no different to any other intelligent and well-run organisation – it creates chains of command. These chains of command drastically simplify the organisational system and consist of nodes around which the body organises itself.

The branch of mathematics involved in these connections is known as *systems theory*. Systems theory is now an incredibly important aspect of modern science, permeating everything from biology to cybernetics. The father of systems theory is Ludwig Von Bertalanffy, who had this to say as to its foundation:

> General system theory, therefore, is a general science of 'wholeness'… The meaning of the somewhat mystical expression, 'The whole is more than the sum of its parts' is simply that constitutive characteristics are not explainable from the characteristics of the isolated parts.

The human body is a perfect example of a system where its characteristics are more than its parts – has science ever isolated the cells responsible for a smile? We know it won't because a smile is a product of wholeness – there are no 'smile cells' in the body.

In systems theory, nodes become of immense importance. A node is a point where lines of communication intersect. On Facebook a node would be someone with 10 million 'friends', in town it is the local café, and in motorway networks it becomes 'spaghetti junction'. In the body a node is an embryological point that controls growth, an organising centre (OC).

In the 1930s the German embryologist Hans Spemann showed that these existed. Spemann worked with early embryos and found areas that directed growth. He successfully transplanted these 'organising centres' and in doing so would also transplant their control of embryo growth and development. In effect, he was able to make creatures' heads grow on their backsides! Spemann went on to perform some of the earliest work on cloning. In 1935 he was awarded the Nobel Prize in Physiology or Medicine 'for the discovery of the organiser effect in embryologic development'.

All around the OC the other cells move, grow and differentiate, but the organising centre does that and that alone. Just like in the fictional TV series *The O.C.*, it is a hub of social networking. It is like a reference point, a centre, a beacon of stability. The organising centre organises and controls.

An OC means that instead of all the cells needing to communicate with each other, they can communicate with just one small area. It stands to reason that the OC would have to be found in areas of great change, in fact at the apex of change. As your elbow forms, the cells going towards your shoulder need to form an arm; likewise, the cells going towards the wrist need to know they are forearm. At a certain spot in the elbow there must be cells that are not going either way – they are stationary and all is moving around them. This is the organising centre.

If there was no organisation then some of the cells in the shoulder may get confused and start sprouting fingers, and the ones in the fingers start to make a shoulder joint. In fact, what is remarkable is how infrequently this occurs: the body's ability to organise itself is so remarkable that it innately finds organisation.

However, in rare cases this process does go wrong, and sometimes a drug given in pregnancy causes this. In the most infamous case, thalidomide was given to women with morning sickness. The drug exists in two forms, effectively mirror images of each other. Unfortunately, whilst one was effective at stopping morning sickness, the other caused serious limb deformities and even death. Mostly the limbs were shortened, but they also suffered from extra appendages and deformity. The cause of this has been extensively studied and is thought to be caused by thalidomide's ability to block new blood vessel growth and bind to a protein called *cereblon*. Cereblon is critical in blood vessel growth in limbs and without this protein the limbs are simply starved of blood.[1]

Whilst cereblon is important for limb growth, its presence still does not adequately explain how the cells differentiate their functions. In other words, some cells in the limb become bone, some muscle and some nerve, yet they all start from very similar stem cells. Even in thalidomide's case, the limbs still formed with muscles and nerves and bones. The lack of blood caused these to be stunted but these structures were still present. Something deeper was involved that enabled the structures to remain integral.

In the US TV series *The O.C.*, organisation is maintained through a hierarchical social structure of money, looks and power; but in the body the OC uses morphogens.

Morphogens (Greek: *morpho-* meaning 'shape', *-gen* meaning 'creating') are powerful growth factors released from specialised embryo cells which diffuse out around the other cells. In 1995 another Nobel Prize was awarded, this time to Christiane Nusslein-Volhard, for the discovery of the first morphogen, which she named Sonic Hedgehog after its ability to make prickly bits appear on the embryo. Nusslein-Volhard showed that the relative concentration along the morphogen gradient affects how the cells develop. For instance, cells closer to the morphogen-releasing cell may become muscle, those further away fat cells, and in the middle bone may form.

These morphogens do not use blood to work; they are not hormones. They work purely by diffusion, by moving in the spaces between cells, between tissues, between organs. They are only ever found in incredibly trace quantities in the blood in health – I would posit that in future we may use their presence in the blood as an early marker for cancer.

At some point in development as the embryo gets bigger another OC will have to arise because another, different, change will be needed. In fact, the body is a seething mass of organising centres all cooperating and competing with each other for control of the cells of the body through morphogens.

In the early stages this process will involve simple diffusion, morphogens moving between cells. As the body gets more complex it creates compartments, which are lined by membranes – fascia. Those cells within the compartment will have a shared purpose, whether it is being bone, moving the bone (muscles and tendons) or regulating the bone (kidney). Morphogens acting on the cells within a compartment will have to tell the different cells within the compartment what they should be doing. However, a different message will be needed *between* these compartments to ensure that they don't grow into each other.

Sometimes what triggers the change in cells isn't even a substance: it can be tension, pressure or even the shape into which the cell is growing.

The morphogen theory not only works in theory, it works in practice; scientists use this to manipulate stem cells. It is a theory that beautifully explains how animal development occurs but still requires control of the organising centres. In other words, there still needs to be a 'brain' – a part of the embryo that regulates the organising centres and the amount of morphogens released.

Except that there isn't! It is just as the title of Ted Kaptchuk's seminal work on Chinese medicine states: it is the 'Web That Has No Weaver'.[2] There is no brain, no overall command centre, no government headquarters. The cells just get on and do it.

At this point we reach the boundaries of what embryological science can currently tell us. We simply cannot describe how this immensely complex process occurs solely by using a cascade of chemicals and growth factors. Scientists understand parts of this process to the extent where they can re-grow hearts and other organs from stem cells, but to do this they need to cheat. They take already formed organs, such as a pig heart, and then strip the cells away. What is left is a matrix of connective fibrous tissue, in a way the skeleton of the heart. Then they use this to act as the template for the new heart. The human stem cells are placed into this template and then they intrinsically start organising themselves around it and form a new heart. What scientists do not know how to do is to get the cells to create the organisational skeleton in the first place.

To understand how the body does this we have to move over to a model that relies not, as embryology does, on descriptions of morphogens and cell reactions, but on a mathematical model of systems. A holistic model that works on the interactions between parts rather than the functions of parts.

'Holism' is poorly understood by most doctors, who think it means to ask about people's social circumstances, but holism means that a part only has meaning when put in the context of the whole. Embryologic development is holistic because parts are always being induced by the rest of the body to develop: without the whole they would be lost; they only know their role when put in the context of the whole body.

Holism is greater than the sum of its parts, and that is exactly what embryological development is – the embryo produces something amazing without having anything tell it to do so; it just gets on with it. Its development *is* greater than the sum of its parts.

Holistic models have been described in the mathematics of complexity and chaos theory, out of which emerges the well-known beautiful fractal pictures of the Mandelbrot sets. Although mathematics may seem dull and dry when compared with the wonders of life, the natural world has a crazy mathematical logic. Understanding the mathematical rules of embryological development allows us to understand embryology better, and this mathematics allows us to understand how Acupuncture may work.

The man who first discovered that nature's chaos has rules was Benoit Mandelbrot. He was undoubtedly a mathematical genius who first saw patterns in a random number generator in his IBM laboratory, but then realised that patterns were present everywhere. His genius was not just in seeing this but also in describing the mathematical rules that governed them. In these equations enormous complexity and organisation occur from a simple feedback mechanism:

$$z_{n+1} = z_n^2 + c$$

This equation may seem complicated to a non-mathematician but considering the infinitely complex and beautiful shapes it produces it is elegant simplicity incarnate. Mandelbrot called these shapes *fractals*, in reference to the *fractured* nature of their form.

As Mandelbrot understood, fractals have laws. These equations produce shapes that constantly grow, and as they do this they eventually come back to where they started. Not only that but they feed back on themselves: in other words if you start with z then the result of the equation is fed back in as the new z. These two aspects mean that, just like in nature, things can spiral out of control very quickly. It also means that tiny changes at the starting point can be amplified out of all proportion. These factors combine to account for the complexity that is seen in the natural world.

The reason a butterfly's wing beating in Japan can create a hurricane in Havana is because of this feedback: a tiny vortex at the beginning is exponentially amplified in the system until it creates a radically more powerful, yet almost identical, effect. The chaotic movement of air around a butterfly's wing is a hurricane in miniature. The conditions have to be perfect for a hurricane to occur, but even so it was the butterfly's wing beating that made the difference.

This tiny change is important, because this same principle is at the heart of why sticking minute needles into the body can effect a healing response. The mathematics of chaos theory allows for tiny changes in the right place to become enormous events. In Acupuncture the skill lies in creating the correct change in the correct place.

The equations that emerge from this mathematics are 'holistic' because one part always feeds back into the next – you cannot remove any part without collapsing the whole equation.

The Mandelbrot set is just one example of beautiful order emerging out of apparent chaos. In this case it is a purely mathematical example but scientists know now that the mathematics of flocks of birds in flight, coastlines, ocean waves and almost all apparently random, yet ordered, natural phenomena obey simple mathematical rules.

The body is a natural system that is highly organised: is it fractal in nature?

Fractals by definition require that they demonstrate self-similarity. In other words, as you go in or out of the fractal you eventually get to a place that looks the same as when you started.

Fractals can be seen in the body:

- DNA itself is a fractal, folding back on itself with a double helix structure.[3–5]

- The branching of arteries, arterioles and capillaries look the same at whatever level.[6]

- Lungs produce self-similarity in the same way as a branch of a tree looks like a mini-tree.[5]

- The surface of the brain consists of folds within folds within folds.[7]

- Muscle cells look like small muscles.

- The kidney collecting system in miniature mirrors the big version.

Even the materials the body is made of are fractal: bones are made of crystals, an inherently fractal structure; fat has been described in 'fractal crystal networks';[8] and proteins self-fold to create fractals.[9]

Delving deeper into the body, almost everything seems to be a fractal, and for good reason – it maximises efficiency,[6] but the body itself does not?

When we look at the structure of individual cells they appear like humans in miniature. They have skin (a cell membrane), a heart/brain (nucleus), lungs that respire (mitochondria), livers that make proteins (endoplasmic reticulum) and even stomachs (called vacuoles). These structures in the cells are even called organelles (little organs).

Furthermore, when we scale humans upwards towards a planetary population level of seven billion (still only one-thousandth the number of our cells) we find that humans en masse start behaving like cells too. We self-organise and differentiate.

Just like a person, en masse our actions can be predicted with unerring accuracy: a city falls asleep at night and wakes in the morning; its guts heave with sewage; its roads pulse with the materials that keep it alive. We think we are all individuals but the reality is we behave as one gigantic hive mind. We create organs of agriculture (stomach); medicine, law and defence (immune system); government (brain); arts (heart and mind); and sanitation (bladder and colon). In fact, this is what the ancient text of Acupuncture, the *NeiJing SuWen*, was alluding too when it described the organs of the body in terms of the functions of the State (see Part III).

A being the size of a planet could easily see human society as a single entity with seven billion cells. If he then looked at the make-up of each 'cell' in enough detail he would come to the conclusion that, like everything of the natural world, he was looking at a fractal.

This conclusion is not startling. The solar system and atoms share the same design; our very universe is fractal.

13

The Leonardos and the Perfect Man

Fractals love the 'golden mean'. The golden mean is a number that goes by many names: 'the divine proportion'; 'the golden ratio'; the Greeks called it Phi and used its aesthetic perfection to full effect in the design of the Acropolis; artists approximate to it in 'the rule of thirds'; and Google defines it as 'the ideal moderate position between two extremes'.

Its value is 1.618…

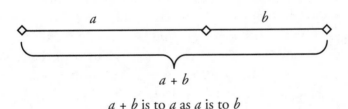

$a + b$ is to a as a is to b

If you want to see a practical demonstration of the golden mean, open your wallet. The rectangular dimensions of your credit cards are no accident: the ratio of length to side is the golden mean.

The golden mean is a ratio that is also found at the end-point of a series of a numbers called the Fibonacci sequence. The Fibonacci sequence was named after an Italian who was called Leonardo de Pisa, but whose nickname was Fibonacci.

The Fibonacci sequence starts at 0, 1 and then the rest of the sequence is formed by adding the last two numbers together:

0, 1, 1, 2, 3, 5, 8, 13, 21, 34, and so on.

The ratio of a number in the series to the previous number gradually approaches the golden mean, or as a mathematician would show it:

$$\frac{1 + \sqrt{5}}{2}$$

What is the relevance of this number?

The golden mean has awed mathematicians, aesthetics and geometrists from the ancient world to the modern. In essence, the golden mean is a way of packing as much into space as possible. Sunflowers use it to maximise their fecundity, and plants use it to ensure each leaf gets as much sun as possible.

The Biomimicry Institute website puts it succinctly:[1]

> Patterning seeds in spirals of Fibonacci numbers allows for the maximum number of seeds on a seed head, packed uniformly, with no crowding at the centre and no 'bald patches' at the edges. In other words, the sunflower has found optimal space utilization for its seed head. The Fibonacci sequence works so well for the sunflower because of one key characteristic – growth. On a sunflower seed head, the individual seeds grow and the centre of the seed head continues to add new seeds, pushing those at the periphery outwards. Following the Fibonacci sequence ensures growth on the same terms indefinitely. That is to say, as a seed head grows, seeds will always be packed uniformly, and with maximum compactness.

As a result of this packing, the golden mean produces perfect spirals where each subsequent turn is 1.618 times as large as the previous, the kind of spirals that are seen in nautilus shells, roses and even galaxies.

One of the most famous spirals of all is seen in DNA and this too exhibits the golden mean. A single cycle of DNA is 34 angstroms* long by 21 angstroms wide. An attentive reader may have noted that these don't just approach the golden mean, these numbers sit *next* to each other on the Fibonacci sequence

---

* An angstrom is one ten-billionth of a metre.

above! DNA displays the ratio of the golden mean because DNA is the ultimate in efficient packing: the secrets of life packed into its tiny spirals.

Our physical body exhibits the golden mean too. Vitruvian man, the famous painting by the other Italian Leonardo, Leonardo da Vinci, purports to show man in his perfect proportions. The ratio of head to umbilicus and feet to umbilicus is the golden mean. The ratios of arm to forearm, hand to forearm, and even the individual bones in our fingers all approach this ratio and, as we shall see, these intersections are where the Acupuncture points are found.

Fractals in nature love the golden mean because the golden mean allows unlimited growth whilst maximising efficiency. If the ratio was higher or lower then growth could still occur but it would be less *efficient*. Spirals would either get too fat too fast, or never really get going. DNA has not chosen this ratio by accident.

DNA itself is inherently fractal too. Those tiny spirals of deoxyribonucleic acid then spirally wind up around themselves to create another spiral in a process that continues on and on. These layers upon layers of spirals are known as DNA supercoiling.

The fractal nature of man points towards a simple organisational system to the body since fractal mathematics is simple. The complexity in fractals arises from the way in which minute changes in the starting position are amplified as it grows. This is just the same as in the fractal of life, where minute changes in the DNA are amplified into all the different species on Earth.

The presence of organising centres and morphogens is what guides this fractal. With indiscriminate use of morphogens there would be chaos, the concentration gradient that guides growth would be disturbed and cells would lose their place. Morphogen theory requires that only certain cells control them, which then maintain their organising power through control over the gradient. The cells need this organising centre, and the organising centres create a network.

How the body creates this network of organising centres is a mystery lost in embryology: it is like trying to describe the mystery of life itself. Genetics may cast some light, but it's going to take a long time because we are talking about relationships between genes rather than the genes themselves. The system it creates is, however, a lot easier to describe.

14

Evolution at
Warp Speed

Your very own human fractal starts from a single cell, for every cell in the body will come from the DNA of this first cell. This simple starting point is rather impressive when you consider that it will create ten trillion cells.

The first cell divides to make two identical cells. These divide again, and again. Now you have eight identical cells. At this point you can remove cells without any harm and make separate embryos. After this the first point of specialisation occurs, the first moment when cells start to take on roles. In IVF this process, known as compaction, is absolutely critical in whether the embryo will survive. The inner cells create a liquid core and the outer cells get tougher. The cells are no longer identical – two different populations have been created.

Fundamentally this split will occur at the level of the DNA. Since the body is being compared to a fractal, this split can be described in mathematical language.

Instead of Mandelbrot's fractal equation:

$$z_{n+1} = z_n^2 + c$$

we have:

$$\text{DNA} + 1 = \text{DNA}^2 + \text{Qi}$$

'DNA + 1' is the little ball of identical cells that have reached a critical mass (+1), which in turn causes a transformation.

The 'DNA^2' represents the two new distinct cell groups, and in each cell group part of the library of DNA has been opened and another part of the DNA has been turned off. Now you have two types of cell but you also have something else, something mysterious, the ability for the cells to work together, intelligent metabolism – Qi.

The activated DNA in the new cells will start to work towards the cells' new purpose. This is healthy and each cell population will continue to divide and develop. Eventually the embryo will get to a point where it will need a new change and this will trigger a new split in the cells. The new cell line will be fed back into the equation. Again, the cell line will split and two new, distinct, populations will emerge. Each cell will have different DNA working within it but the cells will be bound together with Qi.

If this process was drawn it would look rather like an upside down (fractal) tree:

As a result of this process each subsequent cell line will be more and more specialised but also have less and less potential. Using this simple process all 400 cell types in the body are created in precisely the areas they are needed.

The cues that tell the cells to split take many forms, one of which is morphogens; others are electricity, tension and the shape in which the cells are growing.

These splits in cells do not represent simple growth, though: the mathematics of fractals is written in exponentials, not simple addition. To truly be a fractal each split in the cell line needs to be an exponential, an *evolutionary* change.

And of course it is! From an evolutionary point of view, these changes did not take days, months or even years, but more like millions or even billions of years! Just the process of cells deciding to live together in groups took an estimated three billion years and this only represents the first stage of our development. During the process of evolution trillions upon trillions upon trillions of mutations would have occurred in our ancestors' DNA until a sequence appeared that made it into homo sapiens. The nine months that it takes a tiny human to form is 4.5 billion years of evolutionary in fast-forward – a truly stupendous event!

(Or, for those of a creationist bent: God loves fractals!)

It is no surprise then that DNA is written in an exponential language, pairs in a double helix written in base four. After just 150 base pairs of DNA there are more potential combinations than there are atoms in the universe, and human DNA has six billion base pairs!

Each change in DNA that made it into us was a result of an unfathomably large number of 'random' mutations. It is as though Douglas Adams had it right in his book *The Hitchhiker's Guide to the Galaxy*: the Earth is an enormous computer using DNA as its code.

In mathematical terms the body is an enormously well-run and beautiful fractal, and DNA is the source code. Unlike the Mandelbrot set, it does not form endless loops of pixels on a screen but produces endless *Loops of Henle* in the kidney; the spirals in the body are formed not in computers but in the myelin sheaths surrounding nerves; the fractal trees are made in the lung; and the fractal web is woven into neurons in the brain. This fractal program is producing something much more complicated than a picture, in 3D, alive, and it is doing that with information from a strand of fibre one-millionth the width of your hair – DNA.

As a fractal it just keeps going on and on. The history of your DNA stretches in an unbroken line back into the darkest recesses of time and will continue into the indefinite future.

The DNA is the key: it creates the enormous complexity, but it is nothing without the organisational system. The DNA contains all the information but it still needs to be read at the correct place and the correct time. The morphogens are what ensures that this happens, and the genius of this system, the beauty at the heart of the cell, is the way in which the DNA translates these tiny morphogenic messages, these flutters of a butterfly's wings, and turns them not into a hurricane but into the sheer majesty of life. To have done this to the complexity and beauty that we see today has taken a planet the size of the Earth six billion years to perfect.

Life really is a marvel.

And this is where Acupuncture and science merge. For this description of the body involves a fiendishly simple system, a system where organising centres and channels of communication control the body from conception to maturation. The complexity is written into the DNA, but the organisation is fractal simplicity incarnate. And the power behind this organisation is what, in Acupuncture, we call Qi.

15

The Sonic Hedgehog Punch

In peaceful calm, void and emptiness;
the authentic qi flows easily.
Essences and spirits are kept within.
How could illness arise?

NEIJING SUWEN

The organisation of the body uses morphogens to help achieve its aim. What is surprising, considering the immense variety of life, is how few morphogens there are. In fact, every beast in the animal kingdom uses practically the same morphogens because they all develop along similar lines. Sonic Hedgehog may not give a hedgehog its spikes but it is still critical for hedgehog and all other vertebrate development. What changes is the DNA, the source code; this is what gives the variability. The organising centres and the morphogens (Qi) stay fairly constant wherever you go.

What this means is that animals have a system for development. Sonic Hedgehog is a morphogen that organises the brain, muscles, skeleton and lungs. How can something so ubiquitous retain this ability to organise? The answer lies in the nature of the system – Sonic Hedgehog is simply a messenger. When the messenger arrives, the cells know what they are supposed to do – they have been primed by their position in the fractal tree of life, and their DNA awaits activation. In this way Sonic Hedgehog is like the mystical expression of Qi – a substance of health with life-giving properties.

But Sonic Hedgehog is a messenger with power of life *and* death. When it's in the wrong place it causes cancer, just as 'bad Qi' would. Science knows this and has developed medicines that target it. At the cutting edge of medical science sits Vismodegib, a drug that blocks Sonic Hedgehog. This drug cures skin cancer but, in a cruel irony for shareholders, makes almost no money because the surgeons do such a great job with their knives.

In a roundabout way Chinese medicine also attacks Sonic Hedgehog, this time via its gene. It does not do it with cutting edge science, though, but with the shell of a beetle!

The Chinese know this beetle as *Ban Mao* or, its official zoological name, *Myalabris phalerata*. The English know this as a blister beetle, and the compounds that are released include the cantharides.

Ever since first being described in *The Divine Farmer's Classic of Materia Medica* (*Shen Nong Ben Cao Jing*), a collection of medical writings dated to around 200 AD, the Chinese have used this to 'break up congealed Blood' and 'detoxify poison'.[1] Scientists became interested in this because, if you understand the body, 'congealed Blood' and 'poison' sounds like cancer. The molecules they found were named the cantharides, and when they tested them they found they turned off the Sonic Hedgehog gene and induced cell death.[2]

The more we investigate cancer, the more we find that morphogens or morphostats (chemicals that tell cells to remain just so) are implicated. A quick medical journal search[3] of Sonic Hedgehog and cancer brings over 700 results; results that show how this morphogen is implicated in cancer of the pancreas, breast, cervix, stomach, brain…

What these cells are doing is bypassing the normal controls and turning on the Sonic Hedgehog gene to use it for themselves. Cancer is like an out-of-control party where the guests have turned up the music and spiked the punch with Sonic Hedgehog, and then proceed to eat and drink everything before wrecking the house.

Of course, it should be obvious that morphogens are critical in cancer because cancer is a cell that is defying the body plan, and morphogens are the gate-keepers of this. The concept of morphogens being critical to cancer sits just fine with genetics. The genetic model of cancer is that eventually a cell gets so many mutations that it just loses the ability to regulate itself. It stops being interested in being part of the body, and grows recklessly.

Normally, the mitochondria in the cell picks up signals from the body that a cell is in the wrong place or doing the wrong thing and flicks the kill-switch (the *extrinsic pathway* of apoptosis). In this way, rogue cells are always being destroyed. But, for some reason, some cells evade this destruction and become cancer.

As we find more and more morphogen implication in cancer we can come to a new synthesis, a synthesis that not only merges embryology with cancer but also Qi. Cancer isn't powerful because a single cell can overwhelm ten trillion; it is powerful because the body gives it permission to do this through aberrant signalling (or Qi).*

Cancer is the 'disruption of tissue micro-architecture',[5] a failure of morphogen signalling, a failure of Qi. Many cancers in places that can be seen are present in a pre-cancerous stage: cervical cancer starts as cells that resemble skin; skin cancer resembles a mole at the beginning; stomach cancer is preceded by raw irritated mucosa. What is happening with these pre-cancerous changes is that the cells are losing their lines of communication with the body. The medical term for this is *metaplasia*, meaning cells that change their form under stress. The stressors have caused the cells to forget their programming, to lose their connection.

The reason that (for example) smoking cigars gives you mouth cancer is because of the stress on the mouth cells caused by the smoke. The smoke starts to become more of an influence than the body, subtly influencing the cells to change. Geneticists describe this as mutations in the p53 gene or suchlike, but really

---

* The police of this process are the T (thymic) cells of the immune system, whose maturation by neural crest cells is both 'essential'[4] *and* relevant – as we will see in Part II.

the smoking is just being a 'bad influence' (just as your mother suggested). Eventually the cells listen more to the smoke than the body and they completely lose their link with it. This is the beginning of cancer.

It is a funny paradigm because in essence this view of the body sees the cancer cells as being 'possessed' by the carcinogen. Apart from semantics and belief systems there is really very little difference: a carcinogen/evil spirit changes and takes over the running of a cell and turns it against the body. In the case of cervical cancer and stomach cancer this carcinogen is even a living entity – the HPV and helicobacter virus respectively.

We can even eliminate these 'evil spirits' with antibiotics and vaccines and cure the disease. The modern world may feel educated in believing in carcinogens rather than the evil spirits of primitive cultures. Is there any difference?

The main reason for not 'believing' in evil spirits is that these entities all turn out to have names and characteristics. And there are so many that not even Hinduism has enough deities to fight them all.

By understanding these entities we have – since the time of Percivall Pott and his extraordinary observations on scrotal cancer in chimney sweeps – created a new paradigm to cope with this increase in knowledge. This paradigm is called epidemiology – the study of the cause of disease. However, epidemiology does not prove the ancients were wrong; rather, it just shows they were more simplistic.

Simplicity has enormous power, though. The most important event at the Olympics is the 100 metre sprint; water is incredibly common yet so vital; the most valuable things to us are the people we love. In the same way Qi is extremely simple yet very powerful:

> Qi is this intelligent force, the intelligence of knowing what should be where. It is the opposite of disease and the enemy of cancer. When you have strong Qi you defeat cancer.

The incredible thing about this embryological organisational system is that using the word Qi in place of cellular communication creates an almost perfect fit with all that Chinese medicine teaches. Intercellular communication, or Qi, can go backwards and 'rebel', it can become stuck, weak, be congenitally weak, it will have different forms for every organ, you can have external invasions of pathogenic Qi, and lastly it will travel in the channels – the spaces between the cells and tissues.

When Dr Shang devised the Growth Control Theory of Acupuncture he knew it needed to make predictions. The model predicted that these nodal areas would be found to have a high degree of electrical junctions to enable cellular communication – which they subsequently did.[6-9] The model predicted that Acupuncture would cause the body to release growth factors or morphogens – which has also been shown.[10-17] In time, for this theory to be fully proven, Acupuncture will have to be shown to regulate levels of morphogens or morphostats.

What Dr Shang created was a new theory of Acupuncture, so powerful that it can describe the most ancient of therapies yet so up-to-date that it can do so with the most advanced modern knowledge. It described the Acupuncture points not as lines on an inert map of the body but as living bio-energetic nodes in the body, so primal and deep that it should be little surprise that we are only now re-discovering them with biomedical science.

16

What are Acupuncture Points?

How then does this fit in with what we know about Acupuncture channels and Acupuncture points?

There is long historical debate within the Acupuncture community: which were discovered first, the channels or the points? In part, the debate centres on whether the points or the channels are the more important. While some authorities believe it was the channels that were discovered first, since they were documented first, others state that the points are real and the channels have been invented to group them together.

The truth is lost in the sands of time. The ancient texts of Acupuncture are at least 200 years older than the stories of Jesus Christ. They are the oldest known medical canons, and while their survival is testament to the truth within them, it is not even known if these are the first! *The Yellow Emperor's Classic of Internal Medicine* (*HuangDi NeiJing*) dates from the second century BC, but it is known that Acupuncture needles made from bone date from around 1000 years before that.[1]

It is probable that Acupuncture theory is far older even than that. Intriguingly, a fossilised Ice Mummy was found in almost perfect condition at the bottom of a Swiss glacier. He was noted to have strange point-like tattoos on his leg. They called this Mummy *Otzi*, after the Otzal Alps where he was found. When they were published on the internet, an observant Acupuncturist noted that Otzi's tattoos were exactly where he would treat for an arthritic low back, and suggested looking for arthritis in Otzi's back. A CT scan confirmed this.

When researchers systematically analysed these points the results, published in the *Lancet*,[1] were unambiguous:

> a treatment modality similar to Acupuncture thus appears to have been in use long before its previously known period of use in the medical tradition of ancient China (c.1000 BC).

The Iceman was carbon dated to 3200 BC (!), posing the question: 'How ancient is Acupuncture exactly?'

(The second obvious question it poses is: 'What happened to it in Europe?' There is no easy answer to this question, but from personal acquaintances in the Acupuncture community it is easy to see how acupuncturists could be mistaken for witches during the Spanish inquisition.)

Acupuncture wasn't just used in ancient China and ancient Europe. The ancient Mayans, despite having no known connection to China, used thorns from native trees to puncture points on the body that they associated with disease. Whilst little is known about this (this was relayed to me personally by a Mayan descendant in Belize), it appears that the concept of Acupuncture existed in Mayan culture too.

The intuitive truth regarding channels and points is that one cannot exist without the other. To have control you need a messaging system, and a messaging system needs a control centre. The Acupuncture points are the control centres in this messaging system but they would be nothing without the channels of communication. Just like the chicken and the egg it is impossible to imagine one without the other.

The channels exist as conduits for Qi, for what all Acupuncturists must accept functions as intra-cellular communication. The points on the channel are places where this communication gets altered, either through disease or through physiology. A good Acupuncturist knows where this physiology occurs, but more importantly he knows that disease changes this. Therefore, just as there are an infinite number of presentations of illness, so there are an infinite number of points.

What is definitely accepted by all classically trained Acupuncturists is that there are certain places on the body which are considered to be much more powerful than others. These were first detailed in the earliest canon of Acupuncture – the *HuangDi NeiJing* (*The Yellow Emperor's Classic of Internal Medicine*). Found on all the channels in the arms and legs, these are known as the *Shu* points and are named in relation to the flow of water. They are found as follows:

- *Well points:* Beginning of nail on fingers and toes.

- *Spring points:* Next to webbing of toes and fingers.

- *Stream points:* On the wrists and ankles.

- *River points:* Midway along shins and forearms.

- *Sea points:* At the creases of elbows and knees.

It is obvious that all of these points (with the exception of River points) are at areas of great change.

- *Well* points mark the end of the beginning, the start of our nails.

- *Spring* points occur where fingers and toes start.

- *Stream* points occur at the wrist and ankle. Here the large bones of the radius and ulnar break into the bones of the wrist (*scaphoid, lunate, triquetrum, trapezium, trapezoid, hamate, capitate and pisiform*) which lie scattered like pebbles before re-forming into the bones of the hand (the metacarpals) and then into the fingers. Flexor tendons fuse with ligaments to form carpal tunnels, arteries divide and plunge deeper.

- *River* points occur on the shin and forearm.

- *Sea* points are found at the knee and elbow where femur gives way to tibia, radius to ulnar, sciatic to peroneal, brachial to radial, gastroncemius to sartorius, brachioradialis to triceps, and joint cavities reside like great internal seas.

All these points (with the exception of River points) share the same characteristics: they are present at areas of great change. In fact, these points are not just *at* areas of great change, they *are* the areas of great change. These are the organising centres of the arm and leg.

The areas between the points are fairly homogenous: fingers, hands, forearms and arms, one part and another look fairly similar. The difference between them is marked, though, which is why each part has its own name.

The points on the rest of the body follow this simple rule: they are found at places on the body of great change.

On the trunk, the most important points are found in the midline (the *Ren* and *Du* channels), a reflection of the fact that this is the area of greatest change. Then they are found in lines going down the edges of the great muscles of the trunk:

- the linea alba of the *rectus abdominis* (Kidney channel)
- between the rectus and transversus muscles (Spleen channel)
- along the tips of the ribs and edge of the pelvis (Gallbladder channel)
- along the rectus and then up through the nipples (Stomach channel), and
- between the ridges of the back muscles (Bladder channel).

All these lines are the fascial boundaries of the trunk, often distinguished anatomically by thick layers of fascia such as in the linea alba.

The face itself has a relatively high number of points for its small size and these points are concentrated around the ears, nose, mouth and eyes. These are all spots where inside (endoderm) and outside (ectoderm) meet, areas where organisation is critical. These junctions represent the meeting of inner and outer body. On the scalp they are formed in the spaces between bones and the spaces between the muscles of the neck.

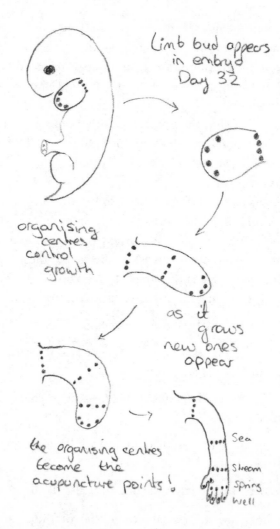

Limb bud appears in embryo Day 32

organising centres control growth

as it grows new ones appear

the organising centres become the acupuncture points!

Sea
Stream
Spring
Well

The classics place very few Acupuncture points in the areas between body contours, and those they do are of less importance. The steeper and more complex the curves in the body, the more change is occurring, the more points will be found. The ear is by far the most complex part of the surface of the body. Look at an ear and notice the curves and complexity within it: for a small part of the body there is a lot going on, so it is no coincidence that the entire ear is littered with Acupuncture points.

The reason these areas have high number of Acupuncture points is because they are not really 'Acupuncture points', they are the embryological organising centres of the body. Even the Chinese word for acupoint (jie 節) translates most precisely as 'node' or 'critical juncture'. The mystery of how Acupuncture works is not a mystery of Acupuncture at all, it is the mystery of growth. Get rid of the organising centres in your elbow and you won't miss the Acupuncture points you have lost, but you will miss your elbow! Likewise with your wrist, ears, jaw and suchlike. The thing that we all take for granted is that these things work, the body self-forms effortlessly, but this is the most amazing thing in existence. There is no overall command centre, it just holistically happens. Compared with 'believing' in this, believing in Acupuncture is easy!

As these embryological control points become mature in the adult, their role is no longer so important because instead of growing the body is now complete. Qi as intelligent metabolism means that it needs to be much stronger when things are developing. This is no different to how an organisation will spend a lot of energy, manpower, brains and dedication to set up a project, but then expect it to almost run itself once done. Animal development is just the same and this is why children can re-grow fingers…they have stronger Qi.

Once humans are mature they need to maintain control rather than install it. Science has coined the term 'morphostats' to describe new chemicals that are used here because the system becomes somewhat senescent. However, it is not that the metabolic energy (Qi) disappears, it is just that it is used for other things… like reproduction.

The facts that Acupuncture points are present at areas of great morphological change, and that these areas of great change require an embryological organising centre, pose more questions about Acupuncture than they answer:

- Why will needling here cause change?

- How can this change be transmitted into the internal organs?

- Why do some points affect the organs in specific ways?

To answer these questions we need to move into the physics of Qi.

17

Currents of Qi

Qi is the organising force of the body. It is intelligent metabolism or, for want of a better expression, the Life Force. It is present in every movement you make, and every breath you take, whether that is of the lungs or the respiration of a single mitochondria.

To make sense of how Qi organises the body we have had to move from mitochondria, through cells, tissues and then into organs. We have had to fast forward through four billion years of cellular cooperation. Even then we still have little idea of how Qi works. We introduce cutting-edge science in the guise of morphogens and understand that cells direct each other through chemical signals. We see that these are controlled by organising centres which spring up spontaneously according to a plan laid down not by any boss but by billions of years of evolution; that the body acts like a 'Web That Has No Weaver'.[1] Finally, we realise that all those spots in the body where there are Acupuncture points are the exact same places where we would expect an organising centre to be.

How does this link in to Acupuncture channels, though? While an organising centre in the elbow may be critical for elbow formation, why should it have anything to do with the heart, or the lung, or any other organ that this most ancient of medicines connects it with?

The body is connected, though! As a doctor I know it is something that Western medics often completely overlook. Medics will argue – po-faced – that the multiple complaints going on in a patient's body have absolutely no relation to each other. It is a ridiculous argument, as what it displays is not erudition but rather a complete ignorance of the connections in the body! The body is connected, the thing that connects it is called connective tissue, and the most ubiquitous connective tissue is fascia.

Fascia is amorphous, it has no real form of its own, but it is everywhere. As stated at the beginning of this book it is completely ignored by Western medicine, and that is why Western medicine completely misses the Chinese concept of Acupuncture.

Qi needs a conduit and what better pathway is there in the body than fascia? It connects and surrounds everything whilst maintaining a completely free pathway between its layers. These pathways of fascia have been detailed beautifully by anatomists, only they were not describing the fascia but the tissues that they enclosed. To badly paraphrase (apologies to Lao Tzu) the ancient Taoist proverb, it is as though they thought:

The space is interesting inside the cup.

If Qi is intelligent metabolism, the Acupuncture points are the embryological organising centres and the channels are the fascial planes which connect these. Then what exactly is being transmitted? Is it just chemicals, morphogens or something more?

The sensation that patients often describe when having Acupuncture is one of an electrical sensation, especially in the limbs. Some points especially create a sensation of tingling or electricity propagating down the limbs. Studies have shown that Acupuncture points conduct electricity better than surrounding skin; that Acupuncture channels conduct electricity better than surrounding tissue;[2] and that channels and points are found in the fascia.[3] From discussion with Dr Wang Ju-Yi and my own practice, I am absolutely certain that the points are found in the fascia. Collagen is the principal ingredient of fascia and collagen has both unusual conducting properties and also generates electricity. Most importantly, the fluid between the fascial planes conducts electricity very well. This fluid is free of any mechanical obstructions…in health.

We accept without any hesitation the reality of our computers working with electricity. The difference between your computer being alive and being dead is often one of software and electricity.

In the same way, death (both heart and brain) is medically defined by the *electrical properties* of the body. Sometimes the hardware (the solid bits) go wrong, in which case you perform a bit of surgery and replace the part. However, often when your computer crashes it is the software, the programming, which is faulty. The software is powered by electricity, which runs invisibly in the computer.

Only a fool would start looking in the computer for where the electricity is stuck or where it is going wrong. We know that it is invisible and only manifests in its effects, so instead we use specialised tools and diagnostics to divine what has gone wrong. We use other computers and electrical devices because these have the required sensitivity. Rocks might work at fixing stuck gears, but are too crude for computers.

Our body is a billion times more complicated than computers and, furthermore, it is not binary in nature; it is quantum or analogue. Emotions are not a black/white affair but are 50-plus shades of grey. When our bodies go wrong then sometimes the only thing that is sensitive enough to pick up on it is something of an equal intelligence and sensitivity – another person. This is one reason behind the 'placebo effect', what has become a sinister catch-all for what is often just 'healing'.

When surgeons are accused of having no empathy it is purely because at one level they need none. A surgeon is a technician and at the end of the day what you want is to have the operation done to the highest technical standard. Given the choice of an excellent technician with poor people skills or a terrible technician with great people skills, I will take the former any day, but that is only because I (somewhat) understand what they are doing. Of course, great surgeons minister to the spirit too, for they understand that it is the spirit that is in charge, not the body. In fact, this ability to empathise is the single biggest predictor of which surgeons get sued, irrespective of technical ability. Surgeons may no longer have the ear of God, but good ones are humble enough to listen.

The problem is that even though computers and humans both have problems with their energy, Western medicine almost entirely ignores this aspect of our reality. The body has this invisible web of energy that connects all parts – it has to in order to grow and function. We can tell when it is wrong because our nervous system brings it to our conscious awareness, but this may be before any physical damage has occurred. The pain is the messenger – not the problem. Instead of using the most sensitive instrument they have (themselves), doctors increasingly rely on machines that measure physical disruption of the body. If your body was a computer then it would be pointless taking it to a doctor with a cold; you would have to wait until that virus had physically started to fry its circuits.

This subtle energy disturbance is important, though. Symptoms are there for a reason: they are a warning sign! Pain is a red flag, your body's attempt to get you to change behaviour. Killing the pain is rarely going to cure the problem, you are just shooting the messenger.

Energy disturbance lies at the heart of all disease; it is the precursor of all disease. Even trauma, apparently the most 'physical' of any disease, is actually simply an issue of excess energy dissipation into the body.

Morphogens and hormones are just a form of concentrated Qi, but there are other factors in the control of the body. The intelligent control system in the body does use morphogens, but I believe that there is also an electrical field that is as important. At the very moment of conception when Yin and Yang, sperm and egg, meet it is electricity that kicks the cell into life. This electricity is intelligent; it carries information; it has Qi; it is not dumb…it is *elecQicity*.

This is the beginning, but this elecQicity persists through the organism's life. ElecQicity is found at every stage of development and in every organism studied.[4] We know that in the very first stages of differentiation – when there are only eight cells – the cells *compact* and form junctions between each other. They use these junctions to communicate with electricity, intelligent electricity, elecQicity. Next the ball of cells forms a liquid internal core, and this change too is driven by an electric current (of sodium ions into the centre).

The currents are tiny and the voltage gradients in the order of millivolts per mm but they are present in the embryology of every organism studied.[4] Furthermore, electricity is involved in regeneration and healing too. Reversing this current causes abnormal development in embryos and abnormal regeneration in animals.[5, 6] Again, this electricity is intelligent – it is *elecQicity*. If we tried to mimic it (for instance, in cloning), we would have to use exact voltages and specific currents to ensure it was right. When we *shock* the heart, we do not do it by connecting the chest to wires coming out of the mains, we use precise currents and in some cases we even synchronise the electricity to the heart's rhythm. We add *intelligence* to the electricity. This is just like how the electrons buzzing around in your computer carry information; that is what elecQicity is – electricity with *biological* information.

Despite the ubiquity of electric fields in our bodies, the research into their effect on growth is still scanty. The West has been more concerned with isolating the growth factors and morphogens – biochemistry rather than biophysics. When we do look, though, we find elecQicity everywhere.

The Chinese knew it was there because as electrical creatures with sensitivity and training we can feel and detect this elecQicity. Acupuncture channels feel different, and points have a different texture. This is unsurprising, as we know they have different electrical characteristics[2] and that we are *Body Electrics*. Trained Acupuncture practitioners and martial artists are sensitive to these forces – they will feel these differences and use them.

One of the most well-respected practitioners of Acupuncture in the UK – Ranald MacDonald – relayed a story regarding this. Studying in China under a Professor of Acupuncture, a sceptical fellow student, a doctor, inquired of the professor:

'But, is Qi real?'

The professor did not answer with words, but instead grasped the lady's hand and firmly pressed on the point *He Gu* (Joining Valley) LI-4. The woman gasped and doubled over in pain.

'You tell me,' he said. 'Is Qi real!?'

His point was made. There is no better physiological explanation for pressure points than using Qi. The proof is as much subjective as anything else: find a reason why pressing in the web between thumb and first finger can incapacitate the strongest of men, and then call that force whatever you want.

If Qi manifests as a form of biological electricity then we would expect it to behave like electricity. We know a lot about electricity because we manage it every day in our modern world and electricity itself behaves in a similar way to water. (*Note*: the following would also be accurate for a morphogen gradient system.)

The ancient texts often compared Qi to water, which is why so many of the point names contain the word *Shui* (water), and why the five main points on the limbs are called Well, Spring, Stream, River and Sea. If they had had the phenomenological recourse to use electricity rather than water I am sure they would have, because electricity provides a much better fit with what they are describing. Water tends to create power through sheer volume, whereas whatever travels in the body is almost invisible. Regardless, water moves in a similar way to electricity:

- It moves from areas of high pressure to low pressure – voltage.

- It moves in a current – amperage.

- It creates power as it moves – wattage.

- Like flowing water it can be isolated (insulated) but will always seek to find a way out and will do this through pathways of least resistance – channels.

- It can bypass things – short-circuits.

In any system with electricity or water (or morphogens) there will be areas of high and low pressure. High pressure occurs in areas where there is much of the substance competing for limited space; low pressure occurs where the substance is able to run freely into space.

In the body the inside will have higher elecQicity than the outside since the outside is essentially void of elecQicity. ElecQicity will move along this gradient, from inside to outside, and it will do so in the pathways of least resistance. The fascial planes provide exactly this – the principle behind keyhole surgery and indeed all anatomical dissection is that these have very low resistance. Fluid in these planes has been found to be rich in ions and an excellent conductor of electricity, and uniquely – apart from the blood – it is completely free of obstructions in health.

It is important to understand that these planes exist everywhere in our body. A hand surgeon dissecting out the small muscles of the hand will move along them, a brain surgeon will move across them to get to the brain, a heart surgeon will work around the fascia of the chest to get to where he wants to go. Fascia shrink-wraps and binds your tissues with a divine attention to detail.

ElecQicity could pass down between the cells in the tissues but there will be more resistance. Unlike with fascia, surgeons have to cut or prise apart these tissues, which resist being separated since they are normally tightly bound together. Surgeons will not do this unless they have arrived at where they want to be…or pathology has forced them to. Surgeons are not making these routes, though; they are just following the plan of the body that God laid down.

Of course, elecQicity needs to enter the fascial compartments to keep the biological communication, and it does, but it does this at the ends of the fascia where one tissue gives way to another. These are the natural spots for the embryological organising centres to be present. Fascia itself is impermeable to almost everything in the body and it is reasonable to assume this is true of elecQicity.

At the end of each fascial compartment sits an organising centre. At this point the energy concentrates but also encounters higher resistance. In the lymphatic system (comprising the fluid which travels in the fascia) these areas are often where lymph nodes are found. Lymph nodes are found at the confluence of these channels of watery lymph to create resistance to filter this fluid. The Acupuncture points are found here too, and it is this combination of high resistance and high energy which means that manipulation here is more powerful. Beyond the organising centre sits another fascial compartment and so the energy moves on.

The elecQicity will have to flow somewhere. High pressure is found internally and low pressure will be found externally. More precisely it will be found at the spots on the body that have the largest surface-area-to-volume ratio since this represents the most external parts of the body. Fingers, toes, ears and nose all share this characteristic and it is no coincidence that all the Acupuncture channels either 'start' or 'end' here.

The elecQicity is generated internally as a way of enabling embryological organisation. It moves in the pathways of least resistance (the fascial planes) and it moves from internal to the external ending in the extremities (fingers and toes).

This is the description of Acupuncture as understood in the East, a description of electrical organising energy, elec*Qi*city running in *channels* that cleave through the body. The West understands these as *morphogens* and *electrical currents* running in *connective tissue planes*.

When the East talks of Acupuncture points, Western embryologists describe organising centres. When the West talks of fascial planes, the East talks of Acupuncture channels.

There is no contradiction in these two views; it is just a question of interpretation. The West may still have no comparable force to Qi, but that is only because it has not attempted to explain the holistic power behind embryological self-organisation.

The channels are not just imagination and manipulation as sceptics would have you believe. They wrap the flesh and blood of our life. The amazing thing, the most incredible fact of all, is that somehow the ancient Chinese seemed to understand connections that we have only just discovered in our most advanced biological laboratories. Somehow these ancient Chinese sages, as humble as the Earth and yet as wise as old turtles, had their ears so close to the ground that they heard the whispers of God. Over thousands of years they compiled this into the most historically consistent medical canons that we have in existence. Somewhere along the way we lost this deeper understanding, only for the mantle to be picked up by the modern magicians of the medical arena – surgeons.

When God forgot to tell surgeons that Acupuncture channels and fascial pathways were the same, was he just playing a joke? Who would have thought Acupuncturists and surgeons share so much common ground?!

The Acupuncture channels of the East are the fascial planes of the West, and when this is understood the enigma of Acupuncture and Chinese medicine cracks open like a walnut shell displaying its perfect centre.

As we shall see in Part II, when fascia and embryology are considered, the Acupuncture channels, essentially unchanged for 3000 years, come into perfect anatomical accord with modern medicine. Within this lies the proof of the argument, for some of these connections are so invisible (see 'The Surfing Channel' in Chapter 28 and Chapter 20 on the Du channel) that we can only see them with the power of electron microscopes, and yet the Chinese described them perfectly.

It turns out that Chinese medicine and Acupuncture is not random, it has a science, and that science is known as embryology. For, when we understand the journey a single cell takes to become the (wonderful, magnificent) creatures we are, we will understand the connections that Chinese medicine teaches.

Part II

The Embryology of
Chinese Medicine

18

An Introduction…
to Yin and Yang

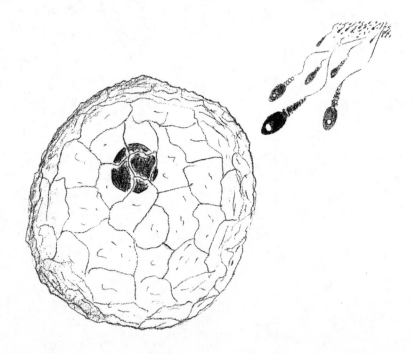

There is a moment before the beginning. It is a moment when a rocket fired by a thousand mitochondria blasts towards a planetary being floating in space. The rocket is in the race of a lifetime; against it are not one but millions of other rockets. Their cargo is a payload of DNA wrapped in an explosive envelope that will blast through into the core of this planet. Here the male and female DNA will combine to create new life. If the rocket succeeds in delivering its payload it will achieve the ultimate prize... immortality.

The world of Yin and Yang is thus shaped. When the Chinese describe the Yang aspects of the cosmos it was male and fiery, rockets and explosions; the Yin was female and earthy, Jane Austen and cream teas.

Yin and Yang form a duality, a completion of the cosmos. In order to understand Chinese philosophy (and hence science) it is necessary to understand this cosmology.

Nowhere is Yin and Yang better expressed than in this ultimate race – the race of sperm to egg. It is difficult to think of a more Yang substance than sperm: it is fast, shaped like a rocket, packed with engines (mitochondria) and even contains an explosive tip.

Yang lives fast and dies young.

Eggs, however, are the archetype of Yin: they are immobile and fat (an egg is thousands of times bigger than sperm), packed with nutrients, but allow themselves to be wafted through life. They are so passive that they just lie there waiting for a sperm to penetrate them, completely incapable even of deciding which sperm will succeed.

Yin barely lives but lasts forever.

Even their origin is a manifestation of the principles of Yin and Yang: sperm are produced on the outside, eggs on the inside.

Yin and Yang do not exist as separate entities, though; they are part of a whole, they cannot exist without each other. When they fuse they complement each other, complete each other, and just as the philosophy of Yin and Yang teaches, start transforming into each other...

The Tao

The One begets the Two.
The Two begets the Three,
and the Three begets the 10,000 things.

TAO TE CHING, CHAPTER 42, 6TH CENTURY BC

When conception occurs, the sperm punctures through the egg with a violence that is immediately felt throughout the cell – it is now impossible for another sperm to enter. This process creates a surge of electricity in the cell: the nuclei combine, fizzing and sparkling with micro-electric sparks.

The cell has done something incredible, it has created new life!
…and then,
just like God at the end of creation…
the cell rests for a day.

A day might not seem like a lot, but in the breakneck world of embryology, it is like a trillion, trillion, trillion lifetimes.

Then it gets to work. It's got three billion years of evolution to get through, and only 12 weeks to do it in! Everything interesting that happens to the baby happens in these 12 weeks; from then until the birth the baby just gets bigger.

The cell starts dividing. This journey it is about to go on is truly the most stupendous journey you can imagine. This cell is going to form you, all ten trillion cells of you.

The first split creates two cells and now these have a one-dimensional relationship – an up and down.

The two cells then divide into four cells. This produces two dimensions of relationships. Now there is an up and down, left and right.

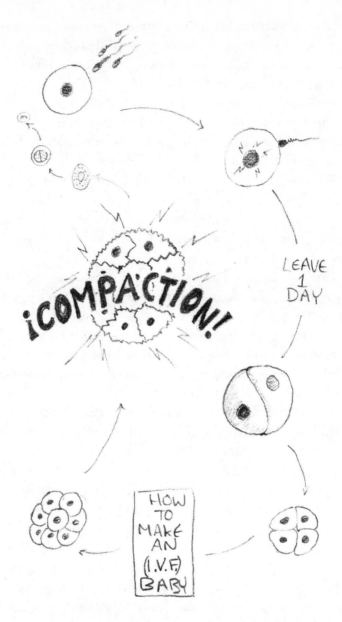

The third split produces eight cells, which add a back and front to the equation. At eight cells there is a ball of cells that have three dimensions of relationships – up, down; left, right; back, front.

It would be tempting at this point to say that this is the beginning of these relationships in our body, that the cell at the 'top' will produce the head, that on the left produce the left arm, and so on. However, our embryology is a little trickier than that. The science of the minute may now be visible on YouTube but it remains horribly complex.

How do these cells go on to form a person?

The first thing they do is *compact*.[1] This means they bind together with electricity like a rugby scrum forming around a ball. The inside becomes softer, the outside harder.*

The compacted ball of cells is still floating at this point. It needs to find a cosy ravine in the walls of the uterus, where it can settle in for the trip of a lifetime. Here it will continue growing.

The embryo is copying our evolutionary blueprint and so, just like every other animal, it forms an egg.

This egg is a bit special, though: it has not one but two 'yolks'. Where these 'yolks' meet it forms, like any two bubbles, a Flat Disc.

This Flat Disc is between the two bubbles. It represents the junction of Yin and Yang; it is the *Taijitu* (more popularly known as the Yin–Yang symbol) in physical form. The two bubbles are called the yolk sac and the amniotic sac.

The yolk sac is so called because it provides the nourishment for the embryo, then brings the blood from the placenta, then forms the future organs of nourishment. The cells lining this sac are called endoderm (Latin: *endo-* meaning 'inner', *-derm* meaning 'skin') and persist as the inner lining of our gut and glands.

In embryological terms yolk is a pretty good match for what the Chinese called Yin. To simplify things, this aspect of the embryo – the yolk sac and its lining of endoderm – I will simply call Yolk.

Attempting to invade and encircle the Yolk is the ectoderm lining of the amniotic sac. (*Ectoderm* means 'outer skin' – which is very appropriate, as we shall see.) We know about the amniotic sac because the baby will swim in this; when a woman's waters burst it is the amniotic fluid from within this sac that leaks out.

---

*   This is possibly the origin of the first two extraordinary channels – the Yin and Yang Wei Mai.

The cells of this sac (ectoderm) encircle the Yolk and in the process create our skin. Furthermore, by a process of *invagination* they make our brain and spinal cord too (see drawing on page 114).

The amniotic sac and the cells lining it (ectoderm) are thus the side of Yang, just as Yolk is the side of Yin. These make the skin which protects us and the brain which controls us; the external and highest aspects of our bodies. These qualities are all Yang in nature.

To simplify things and emphasize how Yang it is (and possibly annoy embryologists to distraction), I will call the amniotic sac and its lining of ectoderm the *Ang*mion.

This junction of Yin and Yang, Yolk and Angmion is where the Flat Disc lies.

(I imagine it looking a bit like how Han Solo, from *Star Wars*, does when frozen in carbonite, although with less detail and bubbling with life.)

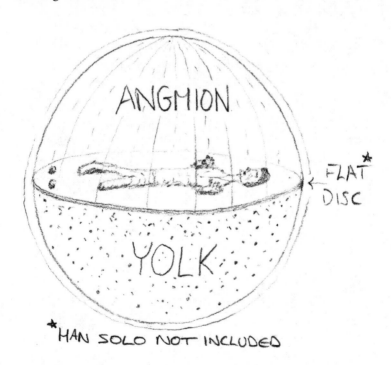

ANGMION

← FLAT* DISC

YOLK

*HAN SOLO NOT INCLUDED

This Flat Disc is where the magic happens. Everything that forms what we know as the baby will come from the cells each side of this disc. Conjoined twins get conjoined at this point; prior to this the split would just form twins.

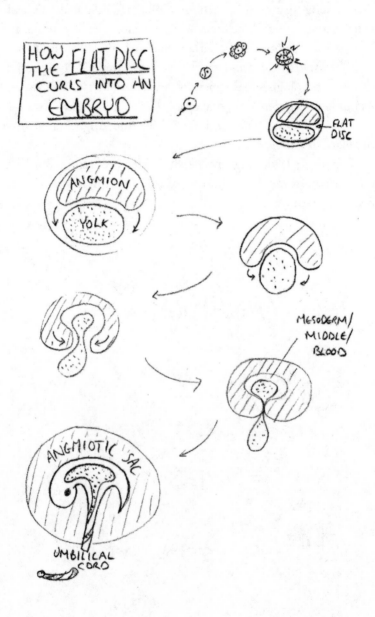

It doesn't stay flat for long, though. Almost immediately the Angmion starts encircling the Yolk.

It is as though a larger balloon is swallowing a smaller balloon by surrounding it. The little tail of the balloon that you can still see becomes the umbilical cord, the little balloon the baby. This is why the baby swims in the amniotic sac.

In between the layers of Yin and Yang, endoderm and ectoderm, another layer forms. This layer is called mesoderm (*meso-* is Latin for 'middle') and forms the muscles, bones, *blood*, parts of the kidney and heart and the connective tissue.

This layer corresponds to what Chinese medicine considers to be Qi (see Chapter 6), or Blood.

The body thus consists of a trinity: the outside, inside and middle; the ectoderm, endoderm and mesoderm; the Angmion, Yolk and Blood.

This trinity is represented in Chinese medicine by the *Taijitu* symbol.

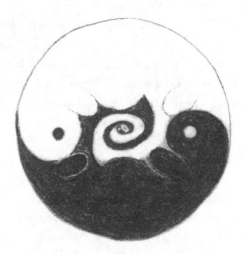

While most people understand this as a duality, many don't realise that there are three elements in this symbol: Yin, Yang and the space between the two. Without this (potential) space, Yin and Yang would not be able to move. This space is considered to be Qi in Chinese philosophy and is the dynamic aspect of the trinity.

The *Taijitu* in fact represents the philosophical evolution from another more primal energy. Earlier drawings of the *Taijitu* are in the form of a spiral, and interestingly the importance of spiral forms can be seen in many other ancient cultures.[2] The spiral energy is seen as the ultimate energy of the Universe in Chinese philosophy.

In Tao philosophy it is said that:

The One begets the Two. The Two begets the Three, and the Three begets the 10,000 things.

The one creates Yin and Yang, Yin and Yang move against each other creating Qi, and these three then produce everything in creation.

The similarity of ancient and modern cosmology is impressive. In the beginning the Big Bang (the One) created matter and antimatter (the Two). Matter and antimatter annihilated each other to produce energy (the Three), and creation was formed.

And in what form is this energy created by the Big Bang?

When we peer into space with our largest telescopes, and inner-space with our most powerful microscopes, we see spirals everywhere. The largest structures that we know of in our Universe are galaxies, and over 60 per cent of galaxies form into spirals. They could have formed into circles, or squares, or any number of shapes, but they created spirals because spiral energy is the basic form of energy, the most primal of energies.

In the '10,000' wonders of creation this spiral energy transforms matter into different shapes and forms but keeps re-emerging, in ferns and Fibonaccis, in whirlpools and whale fins, in nautilus shells and Narwhals' horns. Every single one of us is alive because of a spiral; a double spiral of deoxyribonucleic acid so small that you could fit five billion of them into a single hair. In fact, every living creature on Earth from the giant trees of North America to the tiniest viruses that live in bacteria exists because of this spiral energy.

The largest things in creation and the smallest things of creation bear testament to its power.

The spiral is so powerful a force because it represents two forces with a perfect mismatch; two forces that cannot quite get on, so they move against each other with mathematical exactitude. This mathematical exactitude can be considered another force in itself, and the Chinese called this Qi.

In science they talk about this in the Big Bang – that at the very moment of creation there was 99.999,999 per cent antimatter to 100 per cent matter and that all creation was produced by this reaction, this tiny mismatch between two substances that are otherwise equal but opposite.

Yin and Yang making Qi.

When they re-create these conditions in the particle accelerators in CERN, the futuristic (or primitive?) pictures they produce contain spirals galore.

The formation of the body is no different. When the ectoderm moves over the endoderm to produce the skin, it produces turbulence, and out of this turbulence literally spirals a third type of primitive cell, the mesoderm. This spiralling continues into adult life and is why dermatomes (the way in which the nerves supply the skin) exhibit a spiral pattern.

A note on 'Qi' here. Just as science will talk about electromagnetism as electricity and magnetism (and both) with no apparent contradiction, so the Chinese talk about Qi as a universal force of nature and a more specific force in the body.

Qi allows movement, Qi is movement, Qi is ephemeral…but the body is not ephemeral – the body is solid. In the body the mesoderm forms the space between the inside and outside. Just like Qi, this space is there to allow and create movement and it does this through the heart, blood, muscles and fascia, all of which *do* allow movement:

- The heart moves the blood.

- The blood moves energy and nutrition.

- The muscles move the body.

- The fascia allows the internal organs to slide against each other, and grow against each other.

The third layer (mesoderm) is composed of cells and so this cannot be made of Qi – it would have no material basis; rather it is what is considered 'Blood' in Chinese medicine.

Thus, we have the three layers of the body: the trinity of Angmion, Yolk and Blood. The Angmion protects (skin) and governs (brain), the Yolk nourishes (guts and glands) and the Blood (muscles, fascia and blood) enables movement.

20

Angmion

Beauty and Brains

If we go back to the Flat Disc, we remember that it has two sides. The Angmion side of the Flat Disc is lined with ectoderm, the 'outer skin'. This will envelop the other side to form the outside of your body – your actual skin!

At this point you (or your primitive embryonic beginnings) were about a millimetre in size, or roughly the same size and shape as the comma you just passed. Everything that is going on is occurring in an incredibly precise way.

In the third week of development, on its soon-to-be outside, the Flat Disc does something peculiar.

On either side of its midline it starts to form a wave of cells. These two waves move towards each other and become steeper and steeper as they approach at the midline. Finally, when they meet at the midline they complete each other and form a tube, which completely closes itself off from the amniotic sac.*

This tube of Yang cells burrows inwards becoming the *neural tube*, forming your primitive brain and spine.

As different as they may seem, your brain and skin come from the same place: your brain and spinal cord being the 'skin' cells that buried themselves inside.

Embryology is often deceptively simple, but it can go wrong. The neural tube sometimes doesn't close completely, causing conditions such as spina bifida. In spina bifida there is a little hole in the skin near the bottom that means that the spinal cord is open

---

* That's right, the cells on your back are producing the perfect conditions for embryological surfing…

to the outside. Spina bifida tends to occur near the tailbone, but the tube can stay open anywhere from between the tailbone to the eyebrows (where it is known as craniorachschisis).

So the Angmion forms two main structures:

- the skin

- the spinal cord and brain

plus a strange variety of structures scattered throughout the body that surf off the (neural) tube as it is forming. These are called the neural crest cells and in the dour world of embryology are as cool as a cucumber in a curry.

The Angmion is the primitive cell layer of Yang. Like the sun, Yang is external and of high; it is dynamic and moving. Being masculine it is dominant and controlling! The parts of the body formed by this layer are consistent; they remain the Yang parts of the body. The skin is Yang because it is external, hard and protects. The brain is Yang as it is the highest organ and it controls and governs. These are all Yang qualities.

In Chinese medicine the channel of Yang energy is called the *Du* channel. The word 'Du' has been translated as 'Governing', in the sense of a governor of a province. The actual character is drawn as an uncle and an eye, and represents a respected member of the family keeping an eye on things. Hence the English translation is 'Governing channel' and this is quite a good translation.

The Du channel runs from the anus, up the midline of the back, over the head and then ends at the top lip where it connects with the channel of Yin. When the body was a Flat Disc it would have run up the middle of the ectoderm; when the body becomes a sphere it runs up the middle of the back.

In Western medicine this is the line formed by the neural tube closing in on itself. The way in which the neural tube can stay open causing spina bifida is a demonstration of this channel. When the neural tube fails to close it does this along the exact line of the Du channel – anywhere from the anus to between the eyebrows. The failure to close is because embryological planes have not united –

it is as though the glue between the two sides of the body has not worked, exposing the neural tube to the outside world.

Needling along this line allows access to this plane, and this is how Acupuncture along the Governing channel works.

The Governing channel does exactly that – it governs and regulates the internal organs; unlike the channel at the front, the *Yin* or *Ren* channel, which nourishes. The control that comes out of the spinal cord and brain is not necessary for each organ's survival – they will happily live without a 'brain' controlling them – but it is necessary to tell them how to behave. In the gut these nerves tell it to go faster or slower, in the bladder they tell it to pee or to relax, in the rectum to evacuate, and so on. The brain and spinal cord do govern, and the Governing channel gives access to this at an embryological level of control.

Western medicine uses the Governing channel too. Along the spine the points of the Governing channel are found in between the bones of the back, the exact same points which are used for epidurals and spinal taps. Needles placed here easily and bloodlessly enter into the space around the spinal cord. (Bloodlessly is important: the channels of Acupuncture are bloodless.) Injection of local anaesthetic means that the Governing channel is interrupted and patients who have this done (epidurals) not only lose their sensation to bladder and bowels, they also can't govern them!

21

The Yolk of Our Body

It stands to reason that we have a Yolk – yolks are found in all eggs, and they nourish the embryo. Our bodies are no different since all animal embryos work their way through the same evolution in the first few weeks.

Eventually our Yolk will disintegrate and what persists will form the umbilical cord. As everyone knows, this nourishes the growing baby by bringing blood from the placenta. Until then, the content of the Yolk physically nourishes the growing embryo. But the Yolk does a lot more than nourish – it also creates all the organs for future nourishment.

By about the fourth week the Yolk has become almost completely enclosed by the Angmion, the other side of the embryo. In doing this it turns the Yolk from a sac into a tube. This tube forms the entire alimentary canal, known to most people as the gut, then continues on to return to the umbilical cord via the bladder.

In the process of the Yolk disappearing, the embryo slowly absorbs its contents though the gut and bladder until it completely disappears in the fifth week. This provides nourishment.

The tube formed by the Yolk does not stay simple, though. Near the head it bulges out and grows into the chest and forms the lungs.

The middle part of the tube, where the *12 inches of power* (see Chapter 26) will be found, grows into surrounding tissue to form the liver and pancreas, and becomes the site for the mysterious *Ming Men.*

The lower part loops and bends and folds until it fills the abdomen with guts.

Finally, it curls back up on itself to form most of the bladder before exiting through the umbilicus (belly button).

The Yolk is embryological Yin – the Yin Sac if you like. Yin is associated with nourishment: in Chinese philosophy it is the feminine, maternalistic aspect of our lives.

In the early days the Yolk provides this nourishment; later the Yolk produces all the structures that can create nourishment – it produces the gut and glands that enable goodness to be absorbed from food and it produces the lungs that enable nourishment from the air.

Furthermore, the Yolk is responsible for bringing blood from the placenta, the critical organ of nourishment for the growing baby.

The Acupuncture channel of endoderm and the Yolk is the *Ren Mai* (Yolk Vessel), the channel of Yin. It runs along the front of the body from the mouth, through the urethra, to the anus, joining with the Du channel at each end to form an orbit of the body.

The Ren channel is often translated into English as the Conception channel, but this is a poor translation… Translations of Chinese words are fraught with problems because written 'words' in Chinese are nothing of the sort – they are literally characters! Chinese writing portrays, often complex, ideas through the use of these characters or ideograms. Phonetic-based written languages are literal, but ideograms are much more nuanced. Meanings can overlap and be easily misconstrued.

The character for Ren is composed of two parts. The first character represents a human and the second represents a bamboo with a pail of water at each end: it is a human carrying two large pails of water.

The meaning of this has been translated in various ways: to endure, to supply, to nourish. But in no way does it suggest to conceive. The

Conception vessel is so named because of its clinical importance in conception, not because of its actual function.

It has been mis-named because, rather than conception, what it is concerned with is *nourishment*. In the case of 'conception' this is nourishment of the ovum (the female egg) and the foetus; in the body it is the organs. In fact, in embryological parlance the *Yolk channel* would be a much better name for it, so that's what I'm going to call it.

Acupuncture is the study of energetic lines of connection in the body. These lines of connection run through the lines of least resistance – fascia; and pool in places where change occurs – organising centres. How then does the primitive endoderm, the lining of gut, glands and lung, anchored to the back of our bodies, end up with a channel at the very front of our body?

It's all in the embryology, of course!

When the Angmion encircles the Yolk it leaves a tiny little escape route – the umbilical cord. This umbilical cord plugs into the Yolk as in the drawing.

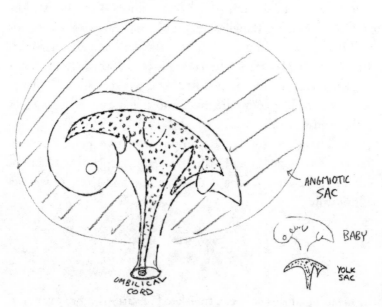

The bit that comes out of the umbilical cord is known as the *falciform* (Latin for 'sickle-shaped') ligament. Everyone has one of these and they rarely cause a problem. This takes blood from the umbilical cord to the heart and sits in the midline, but after birth it almost disappears. This is the connection of the Yolk Vessel above the belly button.

The little outgrowth near the tail is called the *urachus*…

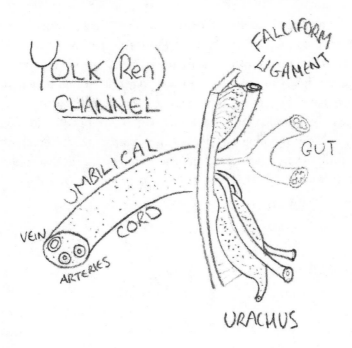

Yikes… I don't like the sound of that… I don't think I'd want to have my urachus go wrong on me…

If you are unfortunate enough to have a urachus gone wrong then it will mean you pee out of your belly button…you really will! It's known as a *patent urachus*.[*]

The urachus connects your bladder to the belly button because it is the remains of the Yolk. This corresponds perfectly with the Yolk channel (Ren Mai) below the belly button and is why Chinese medicine uses many points here for the Bladder (and Kidneys).

---

[*] Thankfully, surgeons can fix this very easily.

Between the chest and the mouth a layer of mesoderm moves in, but there will still be a faint connection. Our body moves and so parts of our body can end up far away from each other even though they started close together. Their fates may be very different even though they started in the same place.

The lines of communication between these cells will remain and the tube of yolk becomes becomes the Ren channel of Chinese medicine.

An analogy is useful. The Yolk channel (Ren channel) is our primitive connection to the innermost aspect of ourselves. This aspect is like a treasure, or a present wrapped in paper. If you wrap a present tightly in paper the only way to get in without tearing the paper is at the edges of the wrapping, even though this is the last place to be wrapped. So it is with us. Tightly wrapped in skin, it is only at the embryological edges of the skin that we can access the most important treasure within. These edges occur at the midline at the front, for this is where the skin (Yang/ectoderm) finally comes together.

22

Blood

The Middle Layer

The mesoderm is the final germ cell layer. It spirals out from the Angmion, occupying the space between the Angmion and the Yolk. The mesoderm creates what many people would consider the body to be: muscles, bones, blood and fat.

Although it produces these it doesn't have the ability to nourish them – that it leaves to the products of the Yolk; and it doesn't have the ability to control and govern them – that it leaves to the Angmiotic sac. Despite this, the mesoderm is still the vast majority of what our body is composed of.

Mesoderm allows movement. On the outside of our body it forms the muscles and bones that move our entire body, it forms the blood vessels and blood that move nutrients and energy, it forms the muscles around our gut and in our diaphragm that move our internal organs, and it forms the muscles of the heart that pump the blood.

Mesoderm also makes the fascia, and the fascia moves the substance of intelligent cooperation – what in Acupuncture theory is called Qi.

Mesoderm forms the kidneys and heart, the axis of our body. The heart is well accepted as the most important organ in embryogenesis and life. In Chinese medicine the Kidneys are seen as equally important to the Heart – they are Yin to the Heart's Yang. The reason for this that is the Kidneys store and are the origin of what the Chinese consider to be one of the *Three Treasures* of our inner life: *Jing*.

Jing

The 10,000

Jing is the fount of our life, the alchemy of Yin and Yang that we inherit from our parents, our constitution. It is the seed of life from which our body springs, flowers and then seeds. This energy is stored within and by our Kidneys,* it creates our body, guides its development, manifests its change into adulthood, and its decline leads us into our old age and senescence.

If there is one thing that you want more of, it is probably Jing. Those (annoying) people in life who can work 18-hour days, spend their lunchtime scaling mountains, and can apparently do this forever without ill-effects, exhibit great Jing. In Taoist thought it is one of the Three Treasures – Jing, Shen and Qi – that need to be nourished for a long life. It is similar to, but ultimately different from, genetics.

Genetics is an amazing science but it has a few flaws, as we now look at.

Genetics is not exact, it can only give you the odds

There is a property of genes called *incomplete penetrance* that (if you'll pardon the pun) is a major pain-in-the-arse for geneticists. It is the reason why geneticists can never give you accurate information about how badly your genes have messed you up.

Incomplete penetrance is almost completely unknown outside of doctors and geneticists but in practice is why someone can have

---

* See 'The Stubborn Organ' in Chapter 25 for explanation of why this is so.

a '57 per cent chance' of cancer when the reality for an individual is either 0 per cent or 100 per cent. It is probably the most important factor in genetics and the reason why genetics will always remain a statistical science.

The difference between what genes you have and what genes you display is about *dominance* (I'm not making this up: geneticists are clearly perverts). Phenotype is dominance, what you see and get, whereas genotype is all the genes you have regardless of whether they are being used. This difference goes some way to explaining why siblings can be so different.

Everybody has at least two genes coding for each attribute, one from the mother and one from the father. When these are the same then the body simply displays the result, like blue eyes. When they are different then the body has to choose one, and so one of the genes becomes dominant. In the example of eye colour then the person can have brown eyes even though they have both blue-eye and brown-eye genes. This is because brown-eye genes are dominant. If the person ends up having blue eyes despite having a brown-eye gene, the brown-eye gene is known as being 'incompletely penetrant'.

Eye colour is simple because it is a single gene coding for the attribute or phenotype, but other phenotypes get much more complicated. In height, for example, there are multiple genes that code for this. Entire genes can be turned off by other genes; this means that even if these are dominant genes, they never get a chance to show it.

The rabbit hole of genetics goes deeper still. Of the six billion bases of human DNA, 90 per cent is considered to be 'junk'.

As genetic science has developed, so too has the understanding that this 'junk' DNA is nothing of the sort. Amongst other things it is thought to prevent bits of DNA working, whilst turning on other bits. DNA is a perfect fractal – smaller units mimic bigger units and the whole thing is folded up upon itself. To enable access to DNA, and hence to allow that DNA to work, it has to be unfolded.

Junk DNA may act more like 'helper' DNA, in the same way that all those components in your computer are vital to help the processor to work.

Junk DNA is not junk at all. Probably, more accurately, our knowledge of junk DNA is junk.

So, even when we know the genetic code we still have major problems. The code itself is unreliable – dominant genes are not always dominant, the genes interplay with each other in ways that are difficult to predict, and 90 per cent of the DNA has functions that are not even understood yet.

Genetics has very little handle on personality

Personality has an enormous effect on genes,* but genes only partly explain people's personalities. Genetic twins with the same genes, the exact same genotype, can end up very different in personalities. Personality is the most subtle, the most ethereal, the most elusive of all things. If personality comes from a subtle expression of genes then it is strange thing, because it feeds back into genes far more strongly: personality is why daredevils risk life, nymphomaniacs pursue sex, and monks become nuns (I'm sure it's happened).

Personality guides the genes to risk themselves en masse, slowly die, or to spread with wild abandon. In studies of identical twins, with the same genes, even the proclivity towards sexual reproduction and sexuality can vary. If one twin is gay, there is less than a 50 per cent chance of the other being gay.[1] If genes were the be-all and end-all of life then you would at least expect them to be decisive in determining whether to procreate!

Ultimately genetics is a very woolly science, which explains why the grand promises and visions of the early genetic pioneers have yet to come to pass. My prediction is that even in 20 years' time we will still have only a rudimentary understanding of how genes create disease.

---

* The 'expression' of genetic characteristics.

If genes can hide and then be coerced into being by something like 'choice', then the science of genetics will have to take this into account. Why some people get diseases and others don't is not just a question of what code they have, but how they are interacting with that code. Study after study confirms that state of mind and health are linked and genetics plays only a part in this. This aspect is talked about in the studies as 'lifestyle' but it could equally be 'personality'.

The Chinese concepts of Jing and Shen are more like this. Shen is personality or spirit and it interacts with our innate strength – Jing. Jing is a substance that is not passive, and in this way it behaves like genes must! Jing is the innate ability of the body to overcome and to prosper.

Jing is a holistic sense of strength, rather than a disparate set of genes. In the film *Gattaca* (named after the bases in DNA – guanine, adenine, thymine and cytosine) the hero of the story is marked down as a genetic inferior but rises above this because despite what the genetic statistics say he has great Jing (also because he has great Shen too).

Genes are statistics; Jing is real.

Chinese physicians do not use genetics to ascertain whether people have good Jing; rather, they look at certain physical attributes of the person. They look at the face to see balance and a strong jaw, they check to see the state of the hair and greying, they ask about teeth and decay and check on the hearing.

What is surprising is that all these physical attributes are produced by a single group of cells. A group who in the dour world of embryology are as sexy as Uma Thurman wielding a sword, or Ethan Hawke blasting into space: a group of cells who are so cool that they even surf…

May I next introduce the surfing stars of embryology: the *neural crest cells.*

Embryological Surfers

Few words have as much power to place dread in the minds of medical students as neural crest cells; with the exception of 'vivas', 'drugs bust' and 'the dean will see you now'.

First, there is their name. To the uninitiated into spangled medicalese it may as well be written in Greek, which of course it is. Neural is Greek for brain tissue, and these cells form at the crest of the incoming waves of cells that will form the neural tube: hence *neural crest cells*.

Second, there is the fact that these are the most dynamic and intriguing of cells – they are the equivalent of supreme embryological surfers. They smoothly and almost effortlessly get into apparently random and wildly separated parts of the body and then perform disparate yet crucial roles.

But! Unfortunately for medical students, unlike the other three layers – endoderm, ectoderm and mesoderm – they appear to have absolutely no logic to what they do.

They have a diversity of function that is both bizarre and vital:

- They form the dentine of the teeth, the layer that is critical for enamel formation, but not the rest of the tooth.

- They form the cartilage, and *only* the cartilage, of the head that will form our facial structure.

- They form the cells that make adrenalin in the kidney (adrenal gland), and they make the conduction pathways and brain of the heart.

- They make the parathyroid glands, hidden deep in the thyroids, a fiddly challenge for thyroid surgeons and their robotic companions.

- They form the support cells of the entire brain and nervous systems.

This makes for fantastic questions in medical exams, questions that surely have no real-life use:

'Does the *sympathetic plexus* emerge from *neural crest cells...* or *mesoderm?*'

Tormenting medical students does not seem to be enough of a reason for their nomadic lifestyle, though, there must be another...

The neural crest cells begin life from the ectoderm, the same part as the brain, spine and skin. When the waves of ectoderm that will form the neural tube meet in the midline the cells at the crest of this wave surf off.

No embryological textbook has ever described them as such, but they really do surf off (inert plastic beads in the same place will find their way to similar places)[1] and not at any time, just as the neural tube is properly *barrelling* up.

The tube is pretty important – it will go on to form the brain and spinal cord – but these cells are far too cool to hang around.

What they do then is unique in embryology. Normal embryological growth is orderly and regimented: morphogens diffuse from organising centres and form orderly lines of growth (see Part I). If cells step out of line and end up were they aren't needed, like good sorts they kill themselves off: this is known as *apoptosis* and – continuing the surfing analogy – is why we have fingers and not paddles.

Neural crest cells, however, ignore this process. They actually move through tissues with impregnability, immune from apoptosis; too cool for school, they just glide into difficult-to-find spots. And they end up at the most important places doing the coolest things, whether it is making the tinniest (sic) bones in our ears, the Schwann cells around our nerves, or the valves of our hearts.

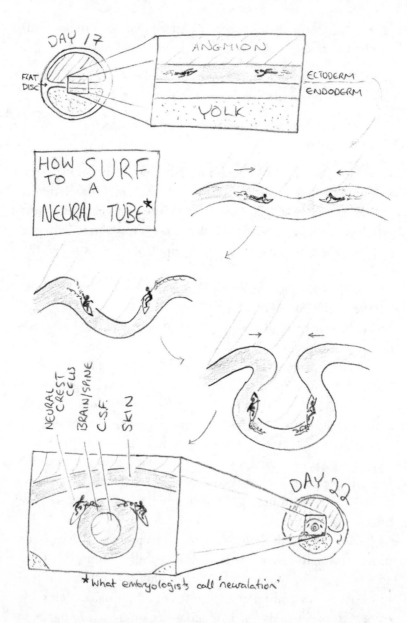

*What embryologists call 'neurulation'

Not only are these tissues widely spaced apart and in very specific areas, they are also universally vitally important. Considering the relatively small amount of body they form they have a massive impact.

In fact, these cells emerged at the point in our evolution when we started to get complicated; they are a manifestation of the intelligence needed to get complicated.[2] Without these cells we would still be jellyfish, or at a stretch trilobites.

This point needs to be emphasised: without neural crest cells we would be primitive invertebrates. Neural crest cells gave us backbones, literally, figuratively and embryonically!

The neural crest cells start off in a thin line in the centre of our back but end up scattered throughout the body with perfect precision. How do they know where they are going and what they are supposed to be doing when they get there?

Who knows? It is a mystery that embryology is still decoding. There are no embryological or fascial planes to explain their movement; instead they appear to divide themselves up and then seek out wherever they need to go.[3] These cells are no surf bums, though – they are instrumental in guiding growth and critical in the formation of organs. For instance, without neural crest cells your heart would be flabby and useless, and your gut wouldn't be able to move.[*]

In a way, what neural crest cells exhibit is great organisational energy or Qi. This strong Qi enables them to create order out of chaos. At an embryological level, strong Qi is a manifestation of Jing.

Strong Jing is reflected in strong teeth, and neural crest cells make these; weak Jing is reflected in going grey and deaf – neural crest cells make the pigment cells and the bones of the ear; Jing manifests in our progression from boy to man, controlled by the pituitary (neural crest help makes this);[4] Jing is exhibited in fine fascial structure and strong jaws, all made by neural crest cells.

The parallels between neural crest cells and inherent strength – Jing – go on, and on. Neural crest cells make the connective tissue of the heart that determines our lifespan, and they are the fire that lights the mythical Ming Men in our duodenum (see the '12 inches of power' section in Chapter 26).

---

[*]   When this happens it is known as Hirschsprung's disease.

Despite the parallels between markers of good Jing and neural crest cells, the former is not the latter. Rather than being Jing, neural crest cells represent the strength of our innate organisational energy. Embryologists describe these cells as the cells that allowed us to get complicated; Chinese physicians described these features as showing strong Jing.

Weak organisational energy will result in neural crest cells that either do not make it or, when they do, cannot function as well. Many of the tissues affected are incompatible with life, but they also include the face, jaw and ear that may be weak or poorly formed. There are at least 700 genetic disorders that involve abnormal facial development alone.[5]

Doctors used to write the acronym FLK for 'Funny Looking Kid' to describe children whose facial features suggested a genetic problem of indeterminate cause. The acronym disappeared the moment patients had access to their notes, but the relationship between facial dysmorphia, neural crest cells and weak Jing remains.

The reason that the Chinese picked up on these markers as showing weak Jing is that these features demonstrate poor organisational energy. The good news for medical students is that it turns out that neural crest cells do have a logic: they represent embryological intelligence, nay, genius! All the wonders of vertebrate life from lizards to birds to mammals manifest their power: the power to create order out of chaos. If this energy is weak then the foundations upon which we are created are weak too.

(When the Roslin Institute got busy with sparks and weird sex (see Chapter 7) the first 276 attempts failed. Those failures did not all end in the test tube. Many animals were produced with too many limbs, and multiple heads. What these mutated clones demonstrated was not abnormal *genetics* (by definition they have *identical* DNA), it was abnormal *Jing* – neural crest cells gone wild – and therein lies a/the difference.)

Neural crest cells are the ultimate intelligence of organisation, and that is why they are good markers for constitutional health problems.

Why do neural crest cells need to do this migration? For instance, the cells surrounding the jaw all contain the necessary DNA to be able to form bone cells but evolution has decreed that these cells are to come from a specific part on the back that creates neural crest cells. Why not the cells that happen to be lying around?

The cells of the conduction system of the heart, the nervous system of the gut and even the cells in the adrenal that make adrenaline all have close links to the nervous system. They all produce nerve cells and neurotransmitters and so it is understandable that they should come from the same stock as the brain.

Why do the cells of the jaw and dentine of teeth, and the bones of the inner ear, go to all the trouble of undergoing this immense and challenging (cellular) migration.

Again, it's all in the evolution!

I'm quite happy to believe that God created us; I just think he did it by placing the ingredients of the world together and seeing what happens. God was an anarchist...no?

Out of this anarchy emerged this amazing order. The order that the embryo uses to grow mirrors the evolution of our primitive ancestors.

All these moves that are seen in neural crest development are critical evolutionary leaps. The facial structure gave us a throat to filter food from air and water, the connective tissue of the heart is vital in how strong the heart becomes, the kidneys change as our embryological development moves from marine to terrestrial.

If God created us in the exact same way as the Bible teaches, then he not only went to all the trouble of faking the dinosaurs, he also went to the trouble of faking the DNA evidence too! What kind of a crazy god is this?

The neural crest cells emerged quite late in evolution, but their existence explains all the wonders of vertebrate life in the world. The pathways they take represent immense evolutionary leaps, logical pathways that appear illogical because they were eked out over millions of lifetimes.

Embryologists may ponder whether they constitute a fourth type of cell, but the Taoists had it better. They got their orders of magnitude slightly wrong, though: the three does not create the 10,000; rather it creates the *10 million* species of vertebrate life in the world.

Neural crest cells occur where organisation and complexity is going through the roof, and the strength of this is what is called Jing.

The Chinese state that Jing is stored in our Kidneys, that the Kidneys create the brain and spinal cord…but to understand why, we have to go into the organs…

Part III

Ming Men and the Six Channels

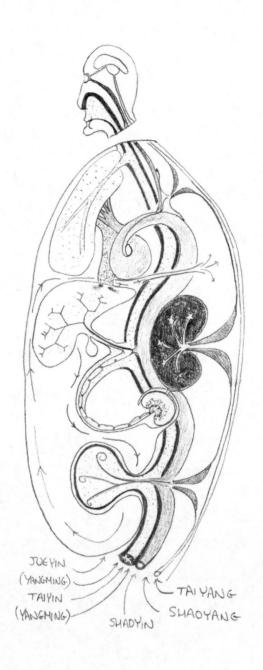

JUEYIN
(YANGMING)
TAIYIN
(YANGMING)

SHADYIN

TAIYANG

SHAOYANG

The Three Yin Channels

The embryo has got to a stage where it is ready for even more complexity (have you?). The one cell turned into many, compacted, formed an egg yolk, made a Flat Disc and then curled that up on itself to form a tiny embryo floating inside an egg.

It has a back and spinal cord; now it must start forming organs. It does this through six great cavities that weave through the body, six cavities that are used as Acupuncture channels.

These six cavities all have a top and bottom, Yang and Yin; and this forms the basis of the Chinese assertion of 12 organs.

Furthermore, the six cavities arrange themselves from back to front, another manifestation of Yang and Yin.

The arrangement of the cavities in the body creates what the Chinese call the six layers, and as we shall see, amazingly, incredibly, these layers all make perfect anatomical and embryological sense:

- TaiYang
- YangMing
- ShaoYang
- ShaoYin
- TaiYin
- JueYin.

These six layers are shown in the figure on the left.

Why six layers? It is simple a question of combination. The three layers – Angmion, Yolk and Blood – divide into each other.

Yin   When embryologists and anatomists draw pictures of these cavities
         they are sometimes drawn as massive spaces, but in reality there is
         almost no space at all. Just like in the drawing of the *Taijitu*, or an
         unopened supermarket plastic bag, the space between the cavities
         is almost invisible.

         The space is potential space.

         These potential spaces are the channels. The 'organs' pair up
         in the channels:

         • Heart and Kidney in the *ShaoYin* (what Western medicine
           calls *retroperitoneal*)

         • Pancreas, Spleen and Lung in the *TaiYin* (what Western
           medicine calls the *anterior pararenal space*)

         • Liver and Pericardium through the *JueYin* (peritoneum,
           diaphragm and pericardium).

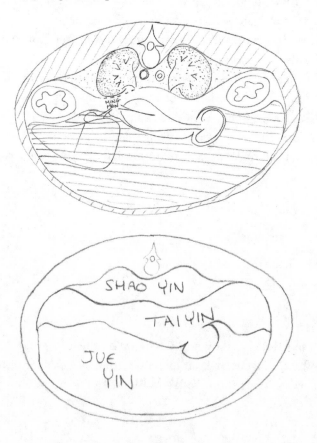

These channels or cavities are known in Western medicine too, *Yin* but in this case they talk about them as *compartments*. As stated in Part I, compartments are like rooms in a house. The walls of the room are made of fascia and the only way in or out is through the windows or doors. The fascia is immensely strong, and just like the walls of your rooms you can't go through them; you have to use the paths in the house.

Your body is like the whole house. Just as in your house, there are connections between all the rooms, including stairs up and down and maybe even hidden doorways (this is the case with Ming Men).

Also just like your house, at one level this arrangement is very simple; there is no need to conceptualise it any deeper. In the same way that you have different roles for the rooms of the house, so does the body, but the house remains its own structure.

These fancy Western names – *anterior pararenal, peritoneal, retroperitoneal* – are just like names of a room – *dining, kitchen, study* – and so the name is not that important. What is important is that they represent a distinct room in the house, a compartment… part of an Acupuncture channel.

This book, and Acupuncture, is about how you move through that house, and the role of each room.

In the same way that you will link your dining room to the kitchen to facilitate ease of eating, so the body also links various organs together.

The Western names listed above have to be included because the whole point of this book is about how Western medicine validates Chinese medicine…all I can do is apologise for the ridiculous names that my fellow doctors have used to describe these compartments…

The organs, and hence the Acupuncture channels, have to connect through the fat layer of muscle between chest and abdomen – the diaphragm. They do this through the only three openings in the diaphragm:

- aorta (Heart and Kidney – ShaoYin)

Yin
- oesophagus (Spleen, Pancreas and Lung – TaiYin)
- vena cava (Liver and Pericardium – JueYin).

Conveniently, the arrangement of these three openings is in the same order as the Chinese place the channels:

- aorta is at the back (ShaoYin)
- oesophagus is in the middle (TaiYin)
- vena cava is at the front (JueYin).

These pathways represent not just the passage of blood and food, but also energy and information.

The correspondence between East and West on this is impressive, but to really understand the channels we have to understand the organs themselves.

The Chinese organs are much more interesting than the Western ones. For starters, they have personalities and they mediate these personalities, appropriately enough, through hormones…

ShaoYin (Lesser Yin)

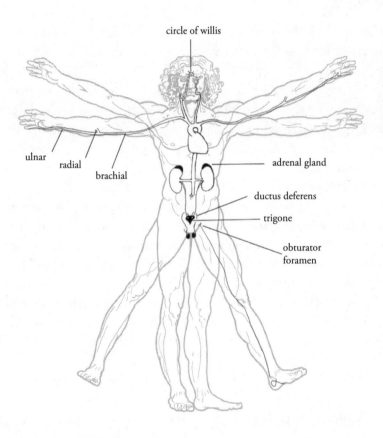

circle of willis

ulnar

radial

brachial

adrenal gland

ductus deferens

trigone

obturator
foramen

Yin

The Emperor

'The Heart is the Emperor, the Supreme Controller'
NEIJING SUWEN, CHAPTER 8, 2ND CENTURY BC

The Heart is the centre of our being. It is here that our emotions live, our hormones beat, where we *feel* our life.

The Heart is the first (proper) organ to appear. Its beating is organised by the nerve energy contained within the cells of the neural crest; it is the manifestation of spirit within matter, Shen within Jing.

The moment our heart stops we die. Our bodies do not carry on living for the few minutes it takes to extinguish our cellular supply of oxygen and glucose; cardiac attack patients do not lie on the floor crying out for help and complaining their heart has stopped.

Why not?

There is a good few minutes' supply of oxygen and glucose in all our tissues, the brain cells should still function, our muscles can still contract, yet the moment our heart stops they die. People who have just had a cardiac arrest should be able to go and call the ambulance themselves!

Cardiac death isn't like that, though; it is instantaneous – it is like a light switch going off. Explaining this away through the physiology of an interrupted blood supply makes no sense…it would take more time.

What happens when the heart stops beating is a catastrophe, not a pump failure.

Chinese medicine has never considered the Heart to be a simple pump, though. The *NeiJing SuWen* states unequivocally:

> The Heart is the Emperor, the Supreme Controller. The Heart is the Fire at the centre of our being, from which Spirit radiates.

Poets and artists have understood this truth for aeons. It was only cold logical science that has denied it the last 400 years. Our literature is full of references to its primacy:

'Follow your heart'

'Listen to your heart'

'A heart-to-heart'

'Have a heart…'

The poets understood the Heart's role at the centre of our being – it is only as we have become more thinking in our culture and less feeling that this has been relegated to a pumping machine. William Harvey's discovery of the Heart as a pump was never meant to dismiss its emotional importance.[1] Thinking occurs in our brain and our Western society is extremely governed by thinking, by deductive reasoning, by logic. Feelings and emotions have been squeezed out as unscientific and fallible. They are anti-scientific, impossible to pin down, irreproducible. One day you like something, the next day not – how can this mean anything?

Western medicine holds that it is our brain that is the centre of our soul. When people commit atrocities we now ask what is wrong with their head, not with their heart. I would argue that in fact it is often their heart where the problem lies. Equally, scientists pore over PET scans and MRI scans of people's brain functions to elucidate where love lies, but I will show that love is only processed in the head, but felt in the heart.

Ironically, it is modern medicine that shows just how important the heart is to our feelings.

The studies on relationships and heart attacks are so dramatic that if you could bottle what occurs between loved ones and sell it as a drug you would be the richest person on Earth.

These studies show that, in fact, one of the most important things for you avoiding a heart attack – along with stopping smoking and exercising – is having a loving relationship![2] Furthermore, if you have a heart attack, forget about getting pills – what you really need is a husband or wife who loves and listens

Yin

to you, for with these people you are three times as likely to be alive after 15 years![3]

Sadly, when your loved ones do die, watch out: broken hearts are real. In the first day after a bereavement people are *21 times* more likely to get heart attacks.[4] There is even a condition called *Takotsubo* cardiomyopathy* that afflicts those with a sudden bereavement and leads to heart failure and death without treatment. Doctors call it 'Broken Heart Syndrome', although this is as likely because they can't pronounce the Japanese as anything else. Strangely, the treatment is the same as for those having a 'real' heart attack, but even in Western medicine, a medicine that has little time for emotions, the cause is accepted to be a broken emotional heart.

Philanderers should be aware too. A recent study shows that men are twice as likely to die of a sudden heart attack with a mistress than with their wife. A cheating heart is also an ill heart.

It doesn't stop there, though. There are now so many case reports of personality changes after heart transplants that many surgeons counsel for this. Stories abound of heart transplant recipients receiving new memories with their hearts, of falling in love with the old flame of their donor, taking up the hobbies of their donor, of developing new tastes that their heart seems to hold, even of changing their sexual preferences from men to women![5]

Yes, these could be coincidences, or side-effects from medication, and that is how they have been dismissed, but it takes a strangely cold person to dismiss stories of hearts that appear to be in love with someone.

There is the touching and heart-breaking story of the mother, a doctor, who could feel her little son's soul in the recipient:

> The first thing is that I could more than hear Jerry's (donor) heart. I could feel it in me. When Carter (the recipient) first saw me, he ran to me and pushed his nose against me and rubbed and rubbed it. It was just exactly what we did with

---

* *Takotsubo* means 'lobster pot' in Japanese because the heart balloons out like one. This is caused by the heart being too weak to physically pump.

Jerry. Jerry and Carter's heart is five years old now, but Carter's eyes were Jerry's eyes. When he hugged me, I could feel my son. I mean I could feel him, not just symbolically. He was there. I felt his energy.

I am a doctor. I'm trained to be a keen observer and have always been a natural-born sceptic. But this was real.

We stayed with the [recipient family] that night. In the middle of the night, Carter came in and asked to sleep with my husband and me. He cuddled up between us exactly like Jerry did, and we began to cry. Carter told us not to cry because Jerry said everything was okay.

My husband, I, our parents, and those who really knew Jerry have no doubt. Our son's heart contains much of our son and beats in Carter's chest. On some level, our son is still alive.

The recipient's mother had this to say:

I saw Carter go to her [donor's mother]. He never does that, he is very, very shy, but he went to her just like he used to run to me when he was a baby. When he whispered 'It's okay mama,' I broke down. He called her mother or maybe it was Jerry's heart talking.

When we went to church together, Carter had never met Jerry's father. We came late and Jerry's dad was sitting with a group of people in the middle of the congregation. Carter let go of my hand and ran right to that man. He climbed on his lap, hugged him and said 'Daddy'. We were flabbergasted, how could he have known him?[5]

Or one young man's father – a psychiatrist – had this to say after his son donated his heart after an accident:

We found a book of poems he had never shown us, and we've never told anyone about them. One of them has left us shaken emotionally and spiritually. It spoke of his seeing his own sudden death. He was a musician too, and we found a song he titled 'Danny, My Heart is Yours'. The words were about

Yin

how my son felt he was destined to die and give his heart to someone.

His donor, an 18-year-old girl, reported:

> When they showed me pictures of their son, I knew him directly. I would have picked him out anywhere. He's in me, I know he is in me and he is in love with me. He was always my lover, maybe in another time somewhere. How could he know years before he died that he would die and give his heart to me? How would he know my name is Danielle? When they played me some of his music I could finish the phrases of the songs.[5]

There is even the tragic case of the 60-year-old who fell in love with the same woman as his donor, and then killed himself in exactly the same way. The poor wife grieved not once, but twice for the same heart.[6]

What these stories relate is *not* coincidence; they are dramatic proof that the heart is more than a pumping machine.

Furthermore, technology now allows the heart to even be replaced by a machine, but at what cost? In Peter Houghton's case, a mechanical pump gradually replaced his failing one over seven years. As a psychotherapist he had a unique insight into the changes this created, and a truly astonishing thing happened: he stopped caring about the people he used to love. He could no longer relate; it literally left him feeling 'coldhearted'. He knew he had grandchildren, he knew he should care about them, but he just didn't, or couldn't, relate to them anymore.[7]

To get to the truth behind the heart's power we have to realise that it is not only an amazing pumping machine, it is also an incredibly powerful electrical generator. In fact, the electrical force that it generates is so easy to measure that physicians do it every time they take an ECG. Being electro-magnetism, this energy propagates outwards at the speed of light. In the time you have taken to finish reading this sentence, the energy from your heartbeat has permeated every living creature on this planet.

We know that people living together become synchronous. Women in communal living find their periods come at the same

time, partners start picking up on tiny cues and finishing each *Yin*
other's sentences, people's body harmonies settle down into a
rhythm (or sometimes they don't and they split apart). The same
is true of people's hearts. Studies of couples show that when in a
state of rapport, of emotional empathy, their heart rates become
matched and that they become mismatched when out of rapport.[7]

When people say that someone's heart is ruling their head it
suggests a person whose feelings are conquering the logic of the
situation. It is often used derogatively, suggesting a person who
is out of touch with reality or who is letting his or her passion
overpower common sense. However, without the ability for our
hearts to conquer logic we would be mere machines, our decisions
left to the cold logic of reasoning.

The great artists, the great love stories, the tales that have
inspired us, none of these would have happened without
surpassing logic. What they all require is exactly that: the heart
has to overpower the head.

Romeo would never have chased Juliet if logic had prevailed;
a mother would have given up on her lost child when all reason
says so; Picasso could never have communicated the impossibility
of art without being illogical.

What these moments of madness have isn't logic – it is
connection. Romeo's connection with Juliet was more powerful
than the logic in his head. He knew the outcome could never
work, his brain processed his feelings thus, but his connection with
Juliet triumphed. His heart ruled his head (this may be a fictional
story but its cultural power arises from its innate truth).

Of course, normally the heart's story is beautiful rather than
tragic. The meeting of a stranger in a bar and the instantaneous
connection that leads to marriage; love at first sight; reunited
family that instantaneously recognise each other; the stirrings that
great art or music produce. This connection is so subtle yet at one
level it is the most real thing that we have.

Despite the primacy of emotion in making us human,
the feelings and connection that this generates still need to be
processed. It is meaningless having this connection if it cannot

Yin   be assimilated into our complex world. Our eyes can see a cup of coffee but it is up to our brains to create all its complex associations – friends, pastries, indigestion and hangovers (not necessarily in that order).

Nobody would suggest that the brain actually sees the coffee; it is up to the sense organs to sense and the brain to process. It is the eyes that see the coffee. The same is as true for our heart as for our eyes. When the author of *The Little Prince*, Antoine de Saint-Exupéry, said:

> It is only with the heart that one can see rightly;
> what is essential is invisible to the eye

he was talking about the heart's ability to sense something more than the physical.

Our hearts 'see' or feel the relationships between each other but leave the head to process the logic of the situation. That is why you can hold two apparently contradictory opinions on somebody; you can love somebody but dislike them. Your heart is linked to theirs, is open to theirs; you love them, but the brain associates them with all the things that you dislike.

This is why the man with the artificial heart felt cold. His brain told him that he should associate his grandchildren with these feelings, it created the memories and the cues for social interaction, but the connection was dead – he (literally) had no heart. Like a blind man cannot see coffee, he could no longer feel relationships.

But we are getting ahead of ourselves. How can the heart even 'feel' someone else?

Matching of emotions and hearts between people is not just a cute example of biological phenomena; it is of pressing evolutionary need. People whose emotions are synchronous should understand each other better and be able to get along, to prosper.

This synchronicity will create patterns, and those patterns will create memories. Memories are neural avenues down which thoughts travel, and they create a basis in physical reality. A neurological imprint.

Yin

The heart's electrical system is neurological in nature. The conducting system of the heart is effectively the same as the brain, relying on the same nerve energy to create its effect. We even have a small brain in our heart built from the cells of the *neural crest*, cells that emerge from the same germ layer as the brain and spine.[8] These will create memory – they will have 'intelligence'.

If one person spends a lot of time with another then the constant interplay of their electromagnetic heart activity will subtly affect each other's hearts.

This last point is a scientific reality. Electromagnetic forces affect other electromagnetic devices. It is why solar flares knock out satellites, or why mobile phones are banned on planes or in hospitals (although the latter is more an example of jobsworths exercising their power than due to any real danger).

Like waves against a rock, these effects may be incredibly faint but they will be there and over time they become stronger and ingrained and form ripples. These ripples will alter the movement of energy in the person's heart and the two hearts will become entwined, their energy will become locked.

In science, the beautiful phrase is *quantum entanglement*: poets call it love.

When your loved one feels something sad or exciting, that change in heart energy will travel as electromagnetic impulses as fast as light. It will move out as waves rippling out from an epicentre. Even before these hit you, your heart will move because if your hearts are in quantum entanglement then this occurs instantaneously! The wave of electromagnetism flowing afterwards will be like a tidal wave of emotion – a solar flare. When your hearts are *in love*, they'll resonate and that is why you know something has happened…

It is not Extra-Sensory Perception; it is Electro-quantum Sensory Perception and it is very, very real (and anyone with a heart knows it).

This is the *Heart* that Chinese Medicine talks about. It is the Heart of Fire, of electricity.

Yin   # Arm ShaoYin – The Heart channel

The Heart emerges from mesoderm, along with the Kidney, and they share the ShaoYin channel, the channel that is rich in blood.

The Heart in Chinese medicine is the organ of Fire within Blood.

It is a fire that starts at the sinus node of the right atrium, moves down the atrio-ventricular node and then fires up the ventricles. It creates so much energy that the electrical impulse travels on, through the aorta and into the arterial system. And it is here, in the aorta, where the Heart channel of Acupuncture begins.

At this point a brief résumé of the embryology of the heart may be informative.

The embryology of the heart begins incredibly simply, but then becomes fiendishly complicated.

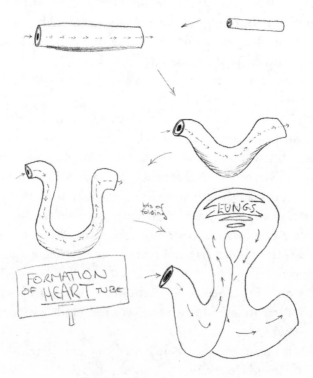

The earliest heart is nothing more than a simple blood vessel that *Yin*
begins to beat. The blood vessel thickens more on one side than
the other, and in doing so begins to take on a U shape, creating a
chamber.

This is the first and simplest fold, but after this the folding that
occurs would test origami masters. It continues folding so that the
blood can be directed from the venous side, through the lungs to
the arterial side of the heart, and then out into the body. This is so
the blood can be energised and cleaned in the lungs.

In order to achieve this the heart creates four chambers, each
with a valve. Things are already complicated, but then it comes
up with some ingenious short circuits that allow the blood to bypass the lungs when the baby is in the womb. The most common
example of this going wrong is an *atrial-septal defect*.

This is why the embryology is so complex, but the important
thing to understand is that in essence the heart is simply a beating
tube.

Well, actually it is two…

The right one pumps blood through the lungs, to be collected
on the other side by the left tube (side of the heart) which pumps
the blood to the rest of the body.

So as a beating tube the heart will only have a single circular
fascial plane with the Qi moving in the same direction as blood:
from the vena cava, through the lungs and then onto the aorta.

The Heart Qi will interact strongly with the lungs. The lungs
are like an upside-down tree with leaves of the finest gossamer,
bathing in a chest full not of air but of gently wafted blood. It's
a slightly crazy visualisation because we tend to have this idea of
the lungs as solid, but the material of the lungs is so fine that it is
blood and air, not lungs, that makes up most of the chest. When
the lungs collapse they occupy no more than a fist-sized space.

This upside-down tree is drawing down air (O_2) and eliminating
stagnant air (CO_2) from the blood. The air is (obviously) vital to
Qi production and in a sense is what the Chinese call Lung Qi.
The Lungs have a closed loop with the Heart enabling blood to be
energised before it will go on to circulate round the body.

Yin   The electrical energy in each part of the heart is insulated. The pericardium prevents it from escaping into the chest, and the connective tissue of the heart prevents it from escaping into other parts of the heart, where it could make the heart beat irregularly. On the left side of the heart the only way out is along the aorta.

Qi movement is all about fascial planes. Like water it moves along the path of least resistance, and in the case of the Heart channel this is along the largest arteries. This begins with the largest artery of all – the aorta.

The arteries consist of three layers that mirror the three layers of the heart:

- The inner layer consists of a thin layer of endothelial cells that forms a barrier to the blood. This is continuous from the heart through the entire vascular system.

- The middle of these layers is more muscular.

- The outer layer is a layer of fascia, continuous with the inner layer of the pericardium that insulates the vessels from the rest of the body.

The fascia in the outer layer will form a continuous barrier between the electrical energy (Qi) of the heart and the rest of the body.

From the heart the Acupuncture channel runs internally to the axillary artery emerging at the armpit. From here it follows the brachial artery to the elbow and then continues down the inner aspect of the arm next to the ulnar artery before finishing at the little finger.

A secondary channel runs up from the heart, along the carotid artery, and then follows the facial artery before ending at the *anastomosis* of fascial and internal carotid artery at the eye.

These, however, are not the descriptions of the Heart channel given in *A Manual of Acupuncture*, Deadman *et al.*'s seminal work on the Acupuncture points,[9] but they are so close as to be practically the same.

His description of the appropriately named first point *Ji Quan* (Supreme Spring) HT-1 advises:

avoid puncturing the axillary artery.   *Yin*

And for good reason, as the point is found right next to it…

Regarding *Qing Ling* (Green Spirit) HT-2, he states that the point is:

> contraindicated in needling by many classics…perhaps because of the danger of damaging the brachial artery.

Too true…

Shao Hai (Lesser Sea) HT-3 is found where the brachial artery splits into ulnar and radial and then the points *Ling Dao* (Spirit Path) HT-4 through to *Shen Men* (Spirit Door) HT-7 are all found directly to the side of the ulnar artery (the description states the tendon of *flexor carpi ulnaris*, but this lies directly above the artery).

I could use arteries to describe any pathway in the body since arteries are everywhere, but the channel is following the principles of Qi physics explored in Part I. It is attempting to flow to the most external along the least resistance (the largest arteries).

(To those anatomists out there: the path to the brachial artery is self-evident, as this is the largest artery. At the elbow the channel follows the apparently smaller artery – the ulnar artery. Why so?

David Kelly, the government scientist, managed to 'kill himself' using the ulnar artery but his was a truly 'unique' and 'exceptional' 'suicide' because this artery is the smaller of the two at the wrist. However, when the brachial artery splits (at *Shao Hai* HT-3) the ulnar artery begins life as the bigger of the arteries before almost immediately splitting to form the *anterior interosseous artery* that supplies the deep muscles of the forearm.

By the time the ulnar artery reaches the wrist it appears smaller than the radial artery, despite the fact it begins life larger. This means that the Heart channel is still following the terminal branch of the largest artery.)

Like water, the Heart Qi will flow to the lowest pressure as quickly as possible. It will do this by flowing down the largest arteries; it won't continue with the aorta into the abdomen since it is attempting to flow to low-pressure areas (as detailed in Chapter 17). This is why the first point HT-1 is known as Supreme

Yin   Spring: the Heart Qi (blood) is bubbling up under pressure from
          below.

          Likewise, Deadman *et al.* describe the accessory Heart channel
          as going to the eye with this description:

> ascends along the oesophagus and then across the face and
> cheek to connect with the tissues of the eye.[9]

Whilst this is no doubt accurate it is probably only because the
common carotid artery also 'ascends along the oesophagus', before
splitting into internal and external carotid arteries. The external
artery then branches off to form the facial artery which 'crosses the
face' and 'connects with the tissues of the eye' where, importantly, it
connects with the ophthalmic branch of the internal carotid artery.

Why it follows this last branch is a mystery, but the fact that
it follows the branch that forms the only connection between the
internal and external carotid artery is extremely important.

This connection (anastomosis) represents a critical juncture
between the supply of blood to the brain and the supply to the
face. Chinese Shen – the strength of spirit – is expressed through
the eyes and the connection between Heart and eyes is paramount.
In Chinese medicine much of what is considered to be the 'Heart',
Western medicine would consider to be under the function of the
brain.

Now, the description whereby the Heart channel flows to the
only connection between the internal and external carotid, face
and brain, does not seem so random.

Like a snail's eye emerging unblinking from its shell, the brain
actually grows into the eye to form the retina. As a result the back
of your eye (your retina) is actually brain, and this is why doctors
look into the back of your eye to see if the brain is swollen!

This mingling between Heart and brain is why the eyes tell
so much about a person, for when you look into their eyes you
really are peering into their soul: that twinkle in their eye is the
nourishment of their mind by their Heart.

Emergency case report

Yin

When describing the Heart channel it was noted that Heart Qi was just following the largest branches. This clearly means that any point with a close connection to an artery will also strongly affect Heart Qi, but in a slightly different way. For instance, it is worth noting that the point next to the radial artery at the wrist is known as the Master Point of the (Blood) Vessels despite it being on the Lung channel. This is consistent with a model of fascial planes, since this point will still maintain a strong connection to the Heart through the radial artery.

The strength of the connection to the heart at this point was tragically illustrated to me as an ER doctor when working in a busy department.

A junior colleague discussed a patient with me: in his 60s, frail and dying of lung cancer, the patient had come in as he was more breathless than normal. The condition was terminal but his family clung on to hope. He was dying, but slowly.

My colleague wanted to do an arterial blood gas – a test to see how much oxygen is in the blood – a test that is coincidentally done at the exact spot of this Acupuncture point. Even when done by experts it is often painful, poorly tolerated, and in this case it would not change the management. It was a pointless test and so I advised her not to do it.

Ten minutes later I was called to a cardiac arrest! The same doctor was there and I recognised the patient as the man with the lung cancer. The ECG showed his heart was flat-lining; there was not even a flicker on the ECG. Desperate attempts were made to try and resuscitate him but the patient had passed away.

The junior doctor was distraught. She told me that she had gone to do a blood gas, fearful that the admitting team would criticise her for not having done one. She had taken the blood from the normal place, at the junction of the wrist and forearm, and gone straight into the radial artery. At the moment she got blood she saw the line on the ECG go flat, and literally the patient died in front of her.

Yin

It is a terrible story, full of heartbreak and remorse… But it illustrates an important point – by having no grasp of Chinese medicine doctors can accidentally do harm. The doctor did cause an iatrogenic death – the medical establishment's term for 'friendly fire' – but Western medicine is unaware why.

This point is most commonly named *Tai Yuan* LU-9, meaning Deep Abyss (!), but unusually it also has two alternate names, one of which is Ghost Heart (!!). The point is also the Master Point of the Blood Vessels – which are controlled by the Heart.

From an embryological/fascial point of view this point has strong connections to the heart through the radial artery. The Qi running along here has a direct connection through the fascia of the arteries to the heart, even though it is on the Lung channel.

When my unfortunate colleague 'needled' here she thought she was just taking a few drops of blood but, in an energetic sense, she drained Qi from the Heart and Lung channels. He was already depleted in both and it was just too much for the dear fellow.

Western medicine is enormously powerful, but it is power that is often aimed with a scattergun approach: this is an example of the dangers of this. Ironically, people like Professor Edzard Ernst have searched with an earnest professionalism for evidence that Acupuncture is dangerous,[10] but the only example in the UK of death by Acupuncture comes not from a traditional Acupuncturist but from a doctor accidentally performing Acupuncture.

All points that have a close connection to arteries thus have a powerful effect on the Heart and should be used with caution, not so much for the risk of puncturing the artery (which is actually quite a tricky thing to do deliberately) but for their action on the heart.

I have had some success massaging the points *Tong Li* (Communicating with the Interior) HT-5 and *Yin Xi* (Yin Accumulation) HT-6 for atrial fibrillation. The nice thing about A&E is you can actually watch the atrial fibrillation resolve on the ECG monitor in front of you! I would highly recommend all practitioners of emergency medicine to know how to find this point and try and use it at the bedside.

The Stubborn Organ

'The Kidney stores Jing and Jing houses our willpower'
NEIJING SUWEN, CHAPTER 5, 2ND CENTURY BC

The heart connects to all the organs through the aorta but it is with the kidney that it has a very special relationship (in both Chinese and Western medicine).

The kidneys and aorta sit in the same space – the retroperitoneum – and this represents the meeting point of the ShaoYin channel.

The Qi from the Heart travels along the largest arteries, going upwards and out to the arms and brain. Downwards the first big branches it finds are the renal arteries, sprouting out from the aorta like two stubby arms, fingers and all. These fingers represent the Kidney function of holding the Qi from the Heart down. At the end of these arms sit two giant beans. They look so like a bean that they have even been named after one – the *kidney* bean!

The picture here is a surprisingly anatomically correct description of the aorta, surprising because it's drawn as a scarecrow:

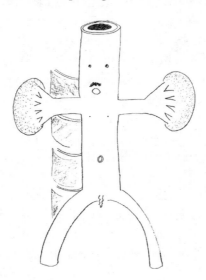

Yin

- The eyes of the scarecrow are the *phrenic (diaphragm) arteries.*

- The moustache is the *celiac axis (stomach artery).*

- The mouth is the *superior mesenteric artery.*

- The nipples are the *testicular/ovarian arteries.*

- The arms are the *kidney (renal) arteries* – holding the kidney beans at the end with their five fingers (branches).

- The belly button is the *inferior mesenteric artery.*

- The scarecrow is male so it has a penis – the *sacral artery*; and two legs – the *iliac arteries.*

- Behind, the scarecrow is attached to a pole (the *spine*) by ropes (the *lumbar arteries*).

Why have I shown you this? It's not to show how clever I am, because the idea is taken from *Anatomy Made Ridiculously Simple,*[11] it's because this picture is so accurate that you can use it for your medical finals…if you need to. Not only are all the positions perfect, but the relative size of the vessels is too.

It's not to help you pass your medical finals either – that's your problem. I showed it because it demonstrates how strong the connection between Kidney and Heart is. The kidney arteries, as you can see, are two broad arms and they need to be: these two little beans take one-fifth of all the blood from the heart!

Chinese physiology considers the Kidneys to not only look like but *act* like two beans too. They are the store of our precious Jing.

We have already discussed how Jing is manifested by neural crest cells. How then does this link with the physical kidney?

The Kidneys are so much more than the physical kidney organ, though.

In Chinese medicine they not only store the Jing; they also 'dominate' water, 'control' the bones, 'fill' the marrow, and are responsible for creating the brain and spinal cord (which are considered to be bones filled with 'peculiar marrow').

The Kidneys are also seen to drive willpower and are the seat
of fear within our body, helping us to manage risk appropriately.

Furthermore the Kidneys are also the basis of our sexuality, the
interplay between Kidney Yin and Yang driving our sexual urge
forwards; as we age this weakening of Kidney energy is why our
sexual drive deteriorates.

Finally, the right Kidney is the abode of the mysterious 'gate
of vitality', the elusive Ming Men.

Before we answer the question of where the channel is, we have
to ask ourselves what were those ancient Chinese smoking when
they wrote all of this?! Is there any way this lot can be reconciled
with Western medicine's view of those little filtration beans in our
loins?

The ad-*Kidney*(?) gland

Chinese medicine has no concept of an endocrinology (hormonal)
system. This is why the organs are capitalised, because the *function*
of the hormone system is linked in with the main organs.

This makes perfect sense really: hormones are messengers
produced by little groups of cells called glands. The messenger
goes everywhere in the body through the blood. It tells other
organs what they should do – speed up, slow down, and so on.
This function is super-important: hormones allow our organs to
tell every other organ what to do in a heartbeat.

In the case of the Kidney, the adrenal gland provides most of
the hormone functions that Chinese medicine talks about.

Fortunately, anatomists have made the connection easy to
make by putting the word 'renal' into this gland. *Renal* is Latin
for 'kidney' and the *ad-* means that it is a bit extra. They called it
this because it sits on top of the kidney, enclosed within it by the
renal fascia. Hence from the point of view of Acupuncture and
embryology it is the same organ, because it shares the same Qi.

The adrenal gland shares not only the renal fascia but also the
renal artery, drains into the *renal vein*, and receives nerve supply

Yin from the *renal plexus*. Linking the ad-Kidney to the Kidney is thus not only a case of etymology but also anatomy. Function follows form and the kidneys and adrenals are part of one system – the adrenals are the messenger system of the kidney.

The adrenal gland is a very interesting gland because it contains the highest concentration of neural crest cell derivatives in thebody.

The adrenal has an inner and outer zone, and it is the inner zone – the medulla – where the neural crest cells surf to. Appropriately enough, this inner zone makes adrenaline, its sister noradrenaline, and a hormone called dopamine. Dopamine is very important in willpower – drug addicts have too little of this in their brain.

When the Chinese state that the Kidneys store our Jing, it is because this gland contains the highest concentration of neural crest cell derivatives in the body. If your neural crest surfing was as good as that of Kelly Slater (11 times world surfing champion), this gland would be in awesome shape.

Adrenaline is very aptly named, coming principally from the adrenal gland. When we are stressed, whether it be by a marauding lion escaped from an inept zoo or a sociopathic boss on the rampage, adrenaline is released by our adrenal gland. It courses through our blood and, as everybody knows, leads to fight or flight. It affects every cell in our body, causing sugar to rush in, mitochondria to go into overdrive and metabolism to speed up. We feel agitated and alert, ready for action. All of these functions Chinese medicine considers to be Yang in nature.

Adrenaline is by far my favourite drug in the Emergency Department. It not only cures asthma and anaphylaxis, but also stops bleeding and bradycardias (very slow heart rates). It is used in tiny doses – micrograms, 0.000,001 of a gram – yet its effects are dramatic and life-saving. It has saved countless lives, my derrière on at least one occasion, and has even changed the course of history – without it Che Guevara would have been beaten by asthma well before Batista's army could try to get to him.

Adrenaline really is an incredible substance. I remember once desperately miscalculating a patient's doubts on whether he was having an early anaphylactic attack. He had been treated in the

past for this in the USA, but seemed unsure whether or not they
were just trying to increase his bill. Seeing no immediate danger
and with a compliant and informed patient we decided to watch
and wait…

Yin

Thirty minutes later he rapidly started turning a shade of purple
best described as puce. His breathing was becoming laboured and
strangely I found myself starting to feel rather unwell. In a cold
sweat I drew up 1 milligram of adrenaline, diluted it 1 to 10 in
water and then diluted this again 1 to 10 in water. What I had now
was 100 micrograms of adrenaline in 10 ml of water.

The patient was feeling very anxious at this stage and said
his heart was racing and felt very unwell – he looked terrible.
Desperately trying to control my own rising heart rate I coolly
reassured him before instilling ½ millilitre – 0.000,005 grams of
adrenaline – into a vein. I waited a few seconds and then infused
another five micrograms.

After 0.000,037 grams I watched in amazed relief as his face
regained its normal colour, his breathing eased, and he said he felt
much better. His anaphylaxis had completely resolved in a matter
of a few minutes, if not seconds! My raging tachycardia took a
while longer…

I learnt a few things that day: don't buy into a patient's doubts
about previous anaphylaxis; tiny quantities of drugs can have
dramatic effects; and adrenaline is a wonder drug.

Adrenaline is a hormone that works on the outside membrane
of the cell, the Yang aspect of the cell.

The cell membrane determines what gets in and out. There are
three ways of getting past the membrane: you can dissolve through
it; you can be admitted through one of the gates on the surface; or
you can send a message through the membrane.

Alcohol does the first, cortisol the second and adrenaline the
third.

Adrenaline attaches to a receptor, remaining outside (Yang)
the cell. Adrenaline never actually enters the cell, being broken
down on the outside. Inside, the activated receptor then turns
on an enzyme that begins a cascade of chemicals, the so-called

Yin

secondary messenger system. This then opens or closes the gates on the outside of the cell to ions and substances, or turns more messengers inside the cell on or off.

In the heart and muscles adrenaline causes extra calcium to enter, increasing strength of contraction; in the lung it causes the muscles to relax, allowing more air in; in the brain it triggers the emotional responses associated with fear.

It is quite incredible how powerful the concept of Yin and Yang is. The Universe does appear to follow this philosophical construct. Adrenaline is not only Yang in its effects, it is Yang in its nature. Yang is external and impermanent, works fast and is aggressive. Adrenaline works on the external part of the cell, incredibly swiftly, and its effects last for minutes to hours rather than days.

If adrenaline is an aspect of Kidney Yang, then what is Kidney Yin in hormonal terms?

The obvious answer is cortisol. Both are produced by the adrenal gland but, embryologically speaking, from two very different parts. Adrenaline, aptly enough, comes from the part that originates from neural crest cells – the Surfers of Embryology – cells which have stealthily moved from the outside of the body to take residence deep inside.

Cortisol comes from the adrenal cortex (this is the origin of its name), an embryological descendant of the mesoderm or Blood layer.

Interestingly, cortisol and adrenaline are often used for the same conditions, the big difference being that adrenaline is used to quickly correct the problem and cortisol is used to correct it more slowly. Again, an example is anaphylaxis.

In anaphylaxis the immune system has decided that a particular substance is a menace and over-reacts. Often this protein is innocuous, such as a nut protein, but sometimes it is genuinely dangerous (like Margaret Thatcher's ideas). Instead of dealing with this proportionately the immune system kicks into overdrive. The body contains mast cells which are supposed to deal with attempted infections: to do this they pump out enormous amounts of histamine and other irritants, which makes the local environment angry and hostile. In anaphylaxis this occurs everywhere and the body itches, swells and goes red. Breathing becomes tight and, if left untreated, the whole process can kill.

As demonstrated, adrenaline is quite the most marvellous cure, but treatment cannot stop there. Adrenaline's half-life is short – a matter of hours – and as it starts wearing off the anaphylaxis returns. The mast cells, which have been switched off by the adrenaline, start to wake up again as the adrenaline is broken down and disappears. The itch and redness can return – rebound anaphylaxis. This is why cortisol is given as well.

Cortisol works very differently to adrenaline. Whereas adrenaline attaches to the outside of the cell, cortisol gets taken in to the very centre – the nucleus. Adrenaline works on whatever is already there, turning proteins on or off, whereas cortisol tells the nucleus to make new proteins or even new cells. Adrenaline works quickly – within seconds – but wears off within hours; cortisol takes hours to work but carries on working for days and days.

Where adrenaline is all the aspects of Yang – outside, impermanent, fast – cortisol is the aspects of Yin – internal, solid, slow.

Cortisol is a drug that used to be given with impunity. In the 1950s and 1960s it was seen as a wonder drug without side-effects. Over time it became apparent that not only were there side-effects but that some of these were extremely serious. The side-effects, however, (as befits a Yin substance) take years to appear (conversely, the side-effects of adrenaline – risk of a heart attack – would appear almost immediately).

The most common side-effects of cortisol include:

- fluid retention

- bone weakening (osteoporosis)

- muscle wasting

- depression and psychiatric symptoms

- high blood sugar (diabetes).

Yin

Yin   In fact, cortisol produces a veritable panoply of symptoms which are another annoyance for medical students. Yet, within Chinese medicine they can simply be seen as a disturbance of Yin function within the body! Cortisol can be seen as draining the body's reserves of Yin to meet an emergency.

Normally in a stressful situation a burst of cortisol would be appropriate and healthy. The cortisol would act to enable the body to cope with this stress by calling on the body's reserves. It would hold on to fluid (Yin) in case the body needed it, it would draw energy and substances from the muscles (wasting) and bones (osteoporosis) to use for vital repairs, it would increase blood sugar to ensure that enough was available, and release white cells from the marrow to enable infection to be fought (but paradoxically make them less aggressive, i.e. more Yin).

Cortisol is doing all these things every day anyway; if our bodies stopped producing cortisol we would become profoundly sick very quickly. The difference is that in times of stress or with drugs this process goes into overdrive.

Cortisol is not Kidney Yin, though; it is an *aspect* of Kidney Yin. There are so many hormones within the kidney that I cannot list them all without getting tedious, but some of them so dramatically prove what the Chinese state that they cannot be ignored…

'The Kidneys dominate marrow'
NEIJING SUWEN, CHAPTER 61, 2ND CENTURY BC

Erythropoietin is a substance produced by the kidney proper. It is best known as the drug of choice for cyclists who like to cheat.

Potent and precise, erythropoietin is released when the kidneys sense low oxygen in the blood flowing through it. The kidney interprets low oxygen as meaning there aren't enough red cells, and releases erythropoietin which travels in the blood to the bone marrow. Here it causes production of red cells. Without this hormone you would get very anaemic, very quickly.

Hence why Chapters 23 and 61 of the *NeiJing SuWen* (*Plain Questions*) states the Kidneys dominate the marrow.

Yin

'The Kidney controls the Bones'
NEIJING SUWEN, CHAPTER 23, 2ND CENTURY BC

Vitamin D is a complex hormone whose production involves the guts, parathyroid gland, skin, liver and kidney. If I tried to describe all these interactions I would have only confused myself more by the end of the chapter. It is so confusing that by the time that it acts on the bone it isn't even called vitamin D any more – it is called *calcitriol*.

However, the end-point of the transformation of vitamin D is the kidneys, and it is these that have the final say in the levels of vitamin D (calcitriol), the most important hormone for bone health. Vitamin D deficiency is known as rickets and it causes weak and poor bone growth. The kidneys control this process by having the final step. The role of the kidneys in bone formation goes further than this, though: the kidneys are instrumental in maintaining calcium and phosphate metabolism, from which the crystals of bone are formed.

It is quite amazing that ancient Chinese medicine intimately linked these two organs. Ask any student of Chinese medicine about the Kidneys and inevitably their role in bone formation will emerge. They are so intimate that they are in fact considered one organ, the bones being a manifestation of Kidney strength. A doctor of Chinese medicine would treat a person with easily breakable bones on their Kidneys!

The Kidneys are related to Water in Chinese medicine, an association that is easy enough to make as the Kidneys filter water from the blood: when the Kidneys are weak, water accumulates in the body.

The bones are seen as being controlled by this same energy and, in fact, really are living crystals that have been precipitated out of solution. Crystals do this all the time in nature: salt crystals

Yin form from supersaturated brine on ships' ropes; and the pressure
of the earth creates *geodes* filled with quartz crystals. In the body
osteoblasts (Latin: *osteo-* meaning 'bone', *-blast* meaning 'builder')
create these conditions by supersaturating collagen fibres with
calcium and phosphate to create crystals. Together these crystals
give bone its hardness and incompressibility.

When I first encountered this Chinese concept of bones and
Kidneys being linked, and of the bones being a substance borne of
Water, it was perplexing. Bones are hard, water soft! It seemed to
be an association that made no sense. Over time, though, the links
have become so compelling that it seems obvious.

Rather than seeing the bones as the dense, dry and dead things
of skeletons and graves, they should be seen as living crystals.
Crystals that grow and dissolve from solution depending on levels
of vitamin D, calcium, phosphate and cortisol, all of which are
controlled by the Kidneys. Crystals that contain and protect the
magical substance in the marrow which replenishes our blood. The
bones and the Kidneys share the same energy, which is why when
the Kidneys get diseased it causes chronic bone weakening, and
drugs that prevent osteoporosis prevent kidney failure.[12]

Snake venom and Kidney Fire

Yet another hormone that comes from the kidneys is *renin*. Renin
is a hormone that has produced one of the most successful classes
of pharmacological drugs in existence – the ACE inhibitors.

Chances are that if you know anyone with even the mildest
heart disease, they are on an ACE inhibitor. ACE stands for
angiotensin converting enzyme, an essential connection between
kidney and heart that tells the heart to do more work. This
connection is there for good reason: it enables the kidney to tell the
heart that it's not getting enough blood. When the blood pressure
in the kidneys drops, cells in a tiny area of the nephron called the
macula densa respond by producing renin.

The renin travels in the blood to the lung where it activates   *Yin*
angiotensin converting enzyme. This creates angiotensin, a
hormone that makes the blood vessels (angio-)tense, makes the
heart pump stronger and also causes the kidney to hold on to water
via another adrenal gland hormone called aldosterone. The result
is that the blood pressure increases and the kidney is happy again
and stops producing renin.

When this connection becomes pathological, the kidneys
start flogging the heart. The heart works harder and harder but
the kidneys are still not happy. The blood pressure rises and the
heart grows tougher and bigger to try and overcome the extra
stress. Eventually the heart, exhausted, collapses and heart failure
develops.

Why this happens in otherwise well people is a mystery, but
what is known is that interrupting this cycle prevents heart failure
developing, or at least slows it down.

Again, the Chinese were aware of this connection between
Heart and Kidney. In fact they placed this at the primacy of life
itself, Kidney storing our Jing and the Heart housing our Shen
(or spirit). Kidney Water controlling Heart Fire, Heart Fire
invigorating Kidney Yin.

They did not know that the kidney produced a hormone called
renin, or that it acted within the lungs to create another hormone
that caused the heart to stress. They didn't know that this then fed
back into the kidney, via the adrenal, to tell it to hold on to more
water.

Instead they talked about Kidney Fire – Ming Men! – flaring
upwards, damaging the Heart. This description is equally valid;
the difference is that when using herbs and Acupuncture there was
no need to define these terms with any more accuracy. Herbs were
used that 'tonified' Kidneys and 'nourished' Water.

There is no doubt that the great physicians of the Han dynasty
would have marvelled at our modern medicine. These physicians
would have used antibiotics and steroids, surgery and anaesthesia,
as well as their herbs and needles. Equally they would have been
amazed that Western medicine had so precisely isolated the exact

Yin   substance that connects the Kidney Fire through to the Heart via the Lungs.*

They would have been even more amazed when you told them that you had isolated an antidote too (ACE inhibitors)! However, when you told them where you got it from – the venom of a cobra – they probably would have nodded sagely; these were physicians who were used to using all of nature's pharmacopeia.

The kidney affects the heart greatly with its hormones but the heart feeds back into the kidney with equal vigour. Mainly it is through the power of its pumping but there are at least two hormones that the heart produces that affect the kidney – ANP and BNP (atrial natriuretic peptide and brain natriuretic peptide).

This connection through the aorta is special. The power of pumping blood stokes the kidneys in a way that is not found elsewhere amongst the organs. There are at least seven hormones that directly interplay between these two organs (in alphabetical order) – adrenaline, aldosterone, angiotensin, atrial and brain naturietic peptide, dopamine and vasopressin – but despite this, Acupuncture theory teaches that it is the special relationship through the aorta that forms the ShaoYin channel.

Ask any intensive care physician about the body and the organs he is concerned about the most and he'll probably say kidneys and heart. (If he says 'brain' then probe a bit deeper. Intensive care specialists are an intelligent lot and normally are deeply curious; ask them what they do to protect the brain and eventually they'll come round to treating the heart and kidneys.)

When the Chinese describe this as the axis of the body, modern medicine agrees.

'The Kidneys dominate Water metabolism'
NEIJING SUWEN, CHAPTER 61, 2ND CENTURY BC

As well as being a fount of many hormones, the kidney is best known for its ability to clean the blood. Specifically, the kidney removes the water-soluble poisons from the blood.

---

*   The controlling aspect of the Heart in the Ke cycle of Five Elements.

Blood is made of cells, proteins, fats, water…and lots of little things. Fats, cells and to a certain extent the little things are by nature water-insoluble, and these substances leave the kidney in the same shape as when they entered.

Yin

The kidney squeezes the watery part of the blood to extract dilute urine composed entirely (in health) of water and a few ions.

The incredible thing about the kidney is how it goes about making this dilute urine, extracting all the goodness, regulating levels of ions and acid, and then removing the waste products.

In health this process maintains the interior milieu of the body at extremely precise levels:

- Our pH is kept at exactly 7.40.

- Our sodium is kept at 140 mmols/l.

- Our potassium is kept at 4.0 mmols/l.

In order to do this the kidney contains one million nephrons, each of which is a tiny intelligent filtration system.

In embryological terms these nephrons grow out of the mesoderm, the Blood layer of the trinity. This means that they come from the same place as the heart.

This nephron function of the kidney is what in the *NeiJing SuWen* is called 'controlling Water'. The nephrons ensure that there is just enough water in the body and that it contains just the minerals the body needs. It does this by regulating everything within the water, and then allowing osmosis to do the rest.

The water in our body can be seen as a finely tuned cellular bath. If the body needs more water then it holds on to sodium; this causes water to flow back by osmosis. If there is too little calcium for the bones then they metabolise more vitamin D and the nephrons reabsorb all the calcium. If you have a late night and need an Alka-Seltzer in the morning, it is the nephrons which will pee out the excess alkali you have just taken.

The nephrons really do control water, by controlling everything within water. Since water is not only 65 per cent of our body but also an inherently Yin substance, it is logical to state that this

Yin　nephron function of the Kidney is the basis of our Yin energy. Nephron and Kidney Yin are indistinguishable. Anything that damages your nephrons is damaging your Kidney Yin.

When the nephrons fail, they cannot control the solutes in the water, and osmosis results in water 'overflowing' from the Kidneys. The person develops oedema, or water retention, as a result. The *NeiJing SuWen* (Chapter 61) puts the consequences of this very eloquently:

> 'Oedema has its root in the Kidney and manifestation in the Lung.'

This is why renin gets released, to give the nephrons more work. The problem is that if the nephrons are already damaged, this won't help.

As the Kidneys' control over Water weakens then our bodies too become weaker, our skin shrivels and our brains literally shrink within our heads.

'The spirit of the Kidney rules willpower and the survival instinct'
NEIJING SUWEN, CHAPTER 5, 200 BC

The Kidney is not only a source of hormones and the controller of our liquid interior, it is also the seat of our primal state of fear.

All hormones are intimately connected with our state of being, our emotional and psychological health. Hormones released from our organs almost universally function as neurotransmitters too.

Atrial naturietic peptide, adrenalin, vasopressin, serotonin, dopamine, bradykinin, histamine and cholecystokinin are all hormones that you have probably never heard of…but they are all known to have specific effects on the body and these effects often gave them their names.

Serotonin is named because it was discovered when it caused the blood vessels (*sero-*) to contract (*-tonin*), but it is now better known as the happy hormone of Prozac or Ecstasy.

Histamine as a neurotransmitter makes you irritable, but is *Yin*
best known for causing allergic reactions.

A lack of dopamine can cause Parkinson's, but most dopamine
is found in the kidney (adrenal gland) not the brain.

Brain natriuretic peptide is a link between heart and kidneys
that controls the blood pressure, but it is called 'brain' because it
was first discovered as a neurotransmitter.

What is now accepted is not only that all these hormones have
multiple functions, but that they almost all act as neurotransmitters
too. In other words, the hormones are an extension of our brain
and indistinguishable from it – it is as though our organs have
grown out of our brain (or the other way around).

The point where brain ends and body begins is not easily
definable. Even anatomists would agree that the brain, spinal cord
and peripheral nerves are like one, but these peripheral nerves
blend in with the organs. The interface between this tissue and
nerves is blurred: whilst the nerves tell the organs what to do, the
organs produce hormones that equally affect the nerves.

Furthermore, the way in which white cells communicate with
each other involves all the same chemicals and neurotransmitters
as neurons. The white cells behave almost like a mobile brain
network. They have memory (cells) and learn, they communicate
and make decisions, and they adapt and control the body by killing
rogue cells.

The distinction of brain and body, mind and body, has been
created by us but in reality there is none.

Adrenaline is a prime example. It not only makes your heart
race but it also makes you mentally alert and tips you over more
easily into aggression or panic. Almost all the adrenaline in our
body, during fight or flight reactions, comes from our adrenal
medulla, so is that panicky feeling in our brain or our body? When
a claustrophobe becomes panicky because he feels penned in, the
overdrive of his nervous system which results in him sweating,
becoming agitated and his heart racing is coming from adrenaline
produced in the adrenal gland. Often these feelings emerge from
nowhere; there is no conscious awareness of a threat in panic

Yin   attacks. To tell these people that their problem is 'all in the head' is not only insensitive, it is inaccurate. Thinking that the problem is all in the head would be the equivalent of blaming the fire alarm for alerting us to the fire.

When Chinese medicine teaches us that fear is an emotion that is produced and handled by the Kidneys, it appears they are correct.

The sister hormone of adrenaline is dopamine. Science now knows that this is a vital hormone in the brain that regulates risk-taking and willpower. Drug addicts appear to have low levels of dopamine, which makes it difficult for them to control their impulses. Most dopamine in the body is made in the adrenal medulla. In a poetic sense beans and seeds represent the stubbornness of life, the inability to stay lying down. The kidneys' intimate link with dopamine is a reflection of this.

'The Kidney Jing fills the brain...'
GREAT TREATISE OF CHINESE ACUPUNCTURE, ZHANG JIE BIN, 1563–1640

The Kidney controls the Bones, fills the marrow and is the seat of fear in our body. It communicates to the heart through at least five hormones, and does all the stuff that Acupuncture theory teaches. What is still not explained, though, is how the Kidney fills the 'peculiar marrow' in the brain.

In my first medical job I had the dubious honour of being the last ever 'renal houseman' at the Manchester Royal Infirmary, a job that already had been designated as too onerous for newly qualified doctors.

I chose it because I was aware of the importance that Chinese medicine placed on the Kidneys and I liked its coding on the application form – 'A1'. So, I faked a preternatural interest in kidney physiology and they chose me.

It almost killed me – it was back in the days of 80-hour shifts and at one point I worked 212 hours in a ten-day period.

Yin

I remember being so tired that I could no longer understand English: would you want to be treated by a doctor in this state?

With a few honourable exceptions, my fellow renal doctors were vicious uncaring malcontents who had so little life outside of medicine that this sado-masochism gave them meaning. I met a lot of nice people there, though, and one of the senior nurses did say something that has stuck with me ever since:

> 'I don't know if they were stupid before and that's why they got renal failure, or if the renal failure made them stupid, but all the patients with kidney failure *are* stupid.'

She said this with a frankness and honesty that was borne of experience, not prejudice. And she was right! Something was happening in kidney failure that dulled the intellect above and beyond the effect of being ill. The question was: What?

The Kidney has nothing to do with the spinal cord and brain forming, though…or does it?

What we understand as the brain is really two organs in one. Everyone knows the brain is composed of nerve cells; but equally as critical are the support staff that make up the barrier between blood and nerves – the blood–brain barrier.

As usual, the support staff is essential but neglected. Everyone loves talking about their old *grey matter*, but what about glial and Schwann cells, astrocytes and myelin sheaths? When these go wrong you get terrible diseases like multiple sclerosis and epilepsy. All these cells are produced by the neural crest cells and are vital to the brain working.

These cells enwrap the blood vessels and are fastidious about what gets through to the nerves. Nerves are extremely sensitive creatures and the support staff ensure they are well looked after. Scientists are starting to describe this function not so much as a barrier but more as a living dynamic structure – the *neurovascular unit.*

In Chinese medicine the Kidney Jing is seen as 'filling' the brain and this is what keeps the senses alert. It has already been described how Jing and neural crest cells are practically the same; neural crest

Yin cells make the support staff, and so *this* is the connection between Jing and Brain that the Chinese are talking about.

The relationship with the Kidneys *per se* is a little more obtuse. Chinese medicine considers the brain to be bone filled with 'peculiar marrow' (this is not such a crazy description as first sounds – the brain is encased in bone!). Marrow is controlled by the Kidneys and furthermore the Kidneys and Jing are intimately connected.

In the case of the brain, we know that this 'marrow' can un-fill because we can scan the head and find a shrunken brain. My wife (who happens to be a gynaecologist and so only ever sees the head from the bottom of the bed anyway) calls this 'Small Brain Syndrome' which is a much better description than the staid Western description – 'cerebral atrophy'. Brain wasting is, however, the more accurate term.

Brain wasting is practically a universal finding in dementia but is also present in other diseases of the brain. It is always a bad finding, being irreversible, and not a lot is known about it.

Studies show that kidney failure and brain wasting are linked.[13]

There is not a lot more to say about the relationship between Kidney and brain. I am convinced that the Chinese are right, that the Kidney Jing does indeed 'fill' the brain and that this is probably a reflection of the ability of these (neural crest derived) cells to protect the nerve cells within. Wasted brains represent the weakening of Jing as it is exhausted at the end of their lives. However, the science of brain wasting is poorly understood in the West.

'The Kidney energy controls the sex
drive and reproduction'
NEIJING SUWEN, CHAPTER 1, 200 BC

In Chinese medicine, when we ejaculate we expel a little of our power: our Jing. The French call it *le petit mort* and the ancient Chinese Taoists were equally morbid and gave all sorts

of dire warnings about needlessly spreading your seed; they even   *Yin*
prescribed amounts depending on age!

The Chinese keyed this in to a mysterious function of the
Kidney; for the Kidney on the right was the abode of Ming Men:
the most mysterious place in Chinese medicine.

Ming Men has nothing to do with Flash Gordon; it is the
Chinese for 'Gate of Vitality'.

The symbol for gate of vitality is:

命門

The last character is a gate (with two doors). The first character is
more complex: it represents heaven and Earth and more pertinently
the point where the two meet and come out.

Ming Men has many functions and it is more appropriate to
leave a fuller discussion until the '12 inches of power' section in
Chapter 26; however, one of the functions is sexual energy!

The kidneys are intimately linked to sexual energy through
the adrenal glands. The adrenal cortex begins to release sex
hormones (such as testosterone and oestrogen) during puberty
and this continues into adult life. Furthermore, the ovaries and
testes emerge from the primitive kidneys. On the scarecrow at the
beginning of this section you may, or may not, have noticed that
the 'nipples' are the testicular/ovarian arteries, and they start next
to the kidneys because they arise from the embryological kidney.

What this shows is that when the ancient Chinese state that
the Kidneys govern sex and reproduction, they were right! This
is despite the fact that the connections are only evident through
microscopic embryology and hormonal assays, neither of which
were available to medical sages 3000 years ago.

We understand now how the Kidney is more than a filtration
system. It is the controller of bodily water; it is the organ responsible
for healthy bones and of generating healthy bone marrow and
blood; it controls the amount of va-va voom (adrenaline) or rest our
body takes; it stores willpower in the form of dopamine; it forms

Yin a dynamic axis with the Heart through multiple hormones which form the axis of our body; and, finally, it generates the Yin and Yang of our sex hormones and stores the next generation in its loins.

In fact it does everything that the ancient medicine of China has always said it does – it just hadn't been translated into the language of Western gobbledygook.

Chinese medicine says one more thing than Western medicine even acknowledges: it says its Qi runs in the Leg ShaoYin channel.

Leg ShaoYin – The Kidney channel

It is appropriate that the kidney organs, seen as the seeds of our lives in Chinese medicine, resemble two seeds or beans.

Instead of roots, waterpipes drain downwards, and they sit astride the spine giving the impression of sharing a common shoot upwards. The testes also look and act like two seeds, and these also emerge from the embryological kidney.

The concept that form and function can be related like this is common in Chinese culture, but is often belittled by Western science as being primitive. Whilst it is simplistic, it is not necessarily wrong. Walnuts look like the brain and for years in China have been eaten for healthy brain function. Science now shows that the oils in walnuts are, indeed, essential for brain function; they are also very good for testes function, creating strong sperm, and I am sure, in due time, we will find that they are good for marrow health too.

The embryology of the kidney is one of the most peculiar of all the organs, because we have not one but many kidneys. In true medicalese style they are grouped together not in English but cloaked in the mystery of Greek:

- pro-nephros
- meso-nephros
- meta-nephros.

Simply put, these mean First-kidney, Middle-kidney and Ultimate-kidney.

The First-kidney group are, appropriately enough, the first kidneys to emerge, but these are not kidneys as any butcher would understand them. They appear at the stage of life when the embryo is smaller than this comma, there are no organs, and the body resembles a worm rather than a human. These primitive kidneys lie adjacent to each developing worm-like segment and they drain excess waste fluid from around the cells and return this to the Yolk Sac.

These kidneys emerge a full two days before the heart. This doesn't sound like much, but in the breakneck development of our embryos it is the evolutionary equivalent of several hundred million years. Although not a kidney that anyone would recognise, the pronephros truly represents the function of, and hence the Chinese meaning of, Kidney.

The Kidney is so much more than kidney: as we have seen, brain, marrow, bone, adrenals, testes and the even these primitive First-kidneys are all aspects of the Chinese Kidney. In this way the embryology in the 3000-year-old *NeiJing SuWen* is, incredibly, correct – for in Chapter 10 it explains how the brain and spinal cord unfold first (and hence the kidney is the first organ to appear)!

We have to accept that this ancient Chinese medical knowledge of embryology is as bewildering as the stones of Baalbak, the pyramids of Giza or why God only decided to use a spare rib to make women...risqué! The pictures we have of neural tubes forming are made with electron microscopes, not the type of machine that has been found in excavations amongst terracotta warriors in China. This knowledge may have been gleaned from elucidating how we were evolved from more primitive creatures and studying them... Who knows?

The First-kidneys appear as two lines along our primitive back in what will become the neck. The Middle-kidneys continue these lines down the body, with a row of tiny functioning baby kidneys. These drain down into what will become the bladder and perform

Yin

Yin   the function of the kidney until the Ultimate-kidney arrives. These lines and baby kidneys are immensely important for Acupuncture theory as they perfectly explain the position and function of the Bladder channel (see 'The Surfing Channel' in Chapter 28).

Finally, the Ultimate-kidney arises. It grows out of the bladder end of the Middle-kidney and induces the surrounding cells to form the kidney that we all know and love (especially in pie).

The Middle- and Ultimate-kidney are really a continuation of each other, the Middle forming the bladder and the Ultimate the adult kidney. The Middle-kidney also forms the testes and associated piping in the male. The testes start life where the kidneys do, and that's why it drags its arterial supply all the way down into the scrotum.

Ureteric pain (for instance, when kidney stones are being passed) is often felt as going from loin to groin and into the testicles. It is also apparently the worst pain you can get: women who have given birth and have had this pain describe ureteric colic as worse, so any men who have had this pain have the dubious honour of knowing what childbirth is like. Their pain is so classical (extreme and can't get comfortable) that it can be diagnosed from the bedside.

The patients' description of the pain is not 'brain confusion', though (see Appendix 3 for more on the science of referred pain); their pain is simply following the fascial pathways laid down by embryology. These structures all sit along one fascial plane.

This fascial plane starts at the ureter, passes down to the back of the bladder, transfers through the fascia of the prostate, down the *ductus deferens* and ends in the testicles. Pain that lies the other side of the collecting duct embryology (i.e. in a slightly different fascial plane) never follows this pathway – instead it stays as a vague pain in the loin of the back. The reason ureteric pain radiates so far is because it is so intense.

The pain of kidney stones represents the internal pathways of the Kidney to the Bladder, but there are also external pathways. The external pathways are the pathways that lead to the outside, the fingers and toes, and to find these we have to go the fascial Yin coverings of the external kidney.

When the Ultimate-kidney is forming it will have organising centres that tell it where to stop. These organising centres will communicate their messages through pathways, and these pathways will persist in the adult as the fascia. Fascia is – literally and embryologically – the defining aspect of an organ.

The fascia of the kidney wraps it, channels through the *retroperitoneum* to the Heart, communicates with the *bald area* of the liver, and then flows down around the organs in the pelvis… exactly as Chinese medicine has taught the Kidney channel does.

How do we know this?

The kidneys, adrenal glands and vessels are contained within the *perirenal* space which is contained by the kidney fascia.

Qi is not the only thing that flows down fascia; water, air or even blood will, too. Sometimes people can have kidneys that bleed profusely into the kidney fascia itself. When studies are done on where the blood goes, they show that it goes upwards to connect with the bald area of the liver, and it goes downwards to surround the organs of the pelvis.[14, 15]

The upwards connection to the bald area of the liver is one reason why the Kidney and Liver have such a special relationship in Chinese medicine. The other reason is that Kidney Qi flows on the pelvic side of the peritoneum, and Liver Qi flows on the peritoneal side.

The downwards connection takes it over the organs of the pelvis – the bladder, vagina and rectum.

The blood/Qi that flows down into the pelvis surrounds all the organs but doesn't enter them. The dynamic that the Kidney has with the pelvic organs is reflected by this; it shares the *Lower Burner*.

The Qi has to keep flowing onwards, from high pressure to low pressure. It needs a way out of the pelvis and it does this through a little hole called the *obturator foramen* – the only exit of the pelvis. This foramen is exactly where the Kidney channel starts on the leg.

Yin   From the obturator foramen of the thigh the pathway is simply a matter of following the muscular fascial planes of *adductors, semi-membranosus, gastrocnemius, achilles, tibialis posterior* and deep muscles on the sole of the foot.

(*Note*: I spend almost no time on describing the external channels of the body since if the ancients got the invisible/internal channels right, then I'm going to give them the benefit of the doubt when it comes to the visible.)

Up the front of the body the ShaoYin channel continues as the median umbilical ligaments, the remnants of the umbilical arteries. Every umbilical cord should be checked at birth as finding only one artery is a good indicator of heart and kidney disease! (These arteries are visible in the illustration on page 105, either side of the urachus.)

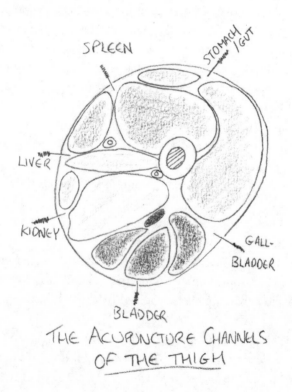

THE ACUPUNCTURE CHANNELS
OF THE THIGH

Emergency case report   *Yin*

The most excruciating medical pain known to man (and woman) is supposed to be kidney stones. In the right conditions, when the urine is supersaturated with calcium, tiny stones form in the kidney. The stones eventually break free and start their tortuous journey down the ureter.

The ureter is not designed to pass stones, it is designed to stop things coming up the other way (such as parasites or bacteria) and as such is very fine. The stones may only be a few millimetres in diameter, but as far as the ureter is concerned it is like trying to pass a baby. (Although I use the word 'stones' I have seen some passed that more resembled Neolithic flint arrow heads!)

The treatment for this is to relax the ureter, to enable the stone to pass. When a woman is passing a baby the body does this with judicious quantities of progesterone and, appropriately enough, a hormone called 'relaxin'! Doctors use painkillers and drugs that block (nor)adrenalin receptors to achieve the same.

The point *Da Zhong* (Large Goblet) K-4 can also be used. It is normally very tender in this condition. This point is a Luo-connecting point so it transfers excess energy from Kidney to Bladder (which is a pretty good description of what a kidney stone is doing!). I'm never quite sure how well this point works as the pain is normally so severe that the patient is always receiving other treatments at the same time.

The Kidney channel is often used in cases of back pain to help support the Bladder channel, especially massage of *Yong Quan* (Gushing Spring) K-1, which lies on the sole of the foot. I've never met anyone who was averse to having this point massaged!

TaiYin (Greater Yin)

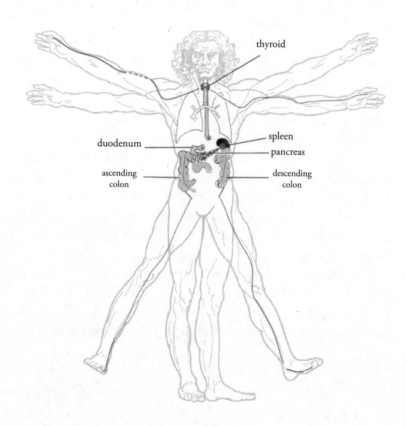

The Inspiring Organ

'The Lung holds the office of minister'
NEIJING SUWEN, CHAPTER 6, 2ND CENTURY BC

To inspire is more than an action, it is a state of being.

Breath is at the centre of our existence, it is the rhythm that sets the pace of our day. Slow and sonorous at nights, gently stirring in the morning, frenetic and laboured as we run for the bus, calm and relaxed as we take our morning coffee. Even the lusty activities of the night are expressed through the lungs.

It is no coincidence that breathing is used in connection to the higher aspects of life. We are not only inspired, but also our spiritual life is intimately linked with breath and hence the lungs. These words share the Latin root *spirare*, to breathe; and this connection between spirit and lungs runs throughout all Latin-based languages. Spirit is considered to be an impermanent aspect of the body, a connection to a higher force, and it is remarkable that the Slavic, Baltic, Chinese and Scandinavian languages also make this connection between this force and the breath. The Hindus, of course, have a long connection through yoga of using the breath to transform the mind and spirit, and as you peruse through all cultures on all continents you will find that the higher, spiritual aspects of society are linked in with chanting, breathing and the lungs.

The lungs are seen as making this connection between body and spirit because they are not only the highest organs in the body but also they deal with the most rarefied of the substances – air. Whilst this connection has little spiritual importance within the world of science and Western medicine, it is of immense importance in our lives. People who lack inspiration are dull and unmotivated. All the greatest inventors, the most intrepid explorers, those who have challenged and changed the status quo, did it because they could

Yin   envisage another world. Without such inspiring people human society would be stagnant. On our own micro-level, finding meaning, purpose and movement in our life depends on our ability to connect with the higher ideals within the world.

If there was one way to describe spirit, suffice to say that there has to be an aspect of life that attempts to rise above the inevitability of death. If we did not have this then the terminal nature of our existence would crush us. It is appropriate that this is linked to air, a substance that rises.

The most important physical function the lungs perform is to exchange carbon dioxide for oxygen, and they do this with a quiet efficiency. When collapsed, the lungs shrink down into a ball the size of a fist, yet if you stretched the surface of the lungs out it would cover a tennis court. The reason such an enormous area can fit into such a small space is that it is incredibly thin. The lungs may be able to be stretched across a tennis court, but it would be $1/200$th the thickness of paper: 500 nanometres thick, a nano-film formed by the original nano-technology – life.

This nano-film forms the leaves in what is in essence an upside-down tree. The trunk of this tree is our windpipe, the branches are the main bronchi, the twigs are the bronchioles and finally the leaves are the alveoli.

The analogy does not end with the physical similarity – they share functional similarity too. Again, nature uses form for function. In the tree the leaves create a huge surface area to enable capture of sunlight and then use it to convert carbon dioxide and water into sugar. In our lungs the alveoli create a massive surface area to capture blood and then convert the carbolic acid stored in it to carbon dioxide and water.

In both trees and lungs the carbon dioxide diffuses in and oxygen is released out (into the blood).

Of course, in the body this process is augmented by many tricks: the haemoglobin has a structure that means it voraciously grabs free oxygen; the thinness of the lining means that the oxygen easily travels across; and the carbon dioxide is saturated in the blood by turning it into carbolic acid – the same thing that makes Coca-Cola fizzy.

Incredibly, the tree uses almost the exact same tricks. The chlorophyll in the leaves has exactly the same structure as haemoglobin – a *porphyrin* ring with a central metal ion. In the case of haemoglobin the ion is iron, in chlorophyll it is magnesium; but the rest of the structure is almost identical! Haemoglobin voraciously traps oxygen, chlorophyll voraciously traps carbon dioxide. The leaves, like the alveoli membrane, are extremely thin to allow oxygen and carbon dioxide to cross.

In the leaves sunlight drives the process; in the body it is spirit.

The twigs, branches and trunk of a tree perform a number of functions that are analogous to the lung. They provide support, carry nutrients to the leaves, and transport sugar and other substances to the roots. Likewise, in the lungs the windpipe and bronchi provide structure to the alveoli, transport the oxygen down to the alveoli and take back the carbon dioxide and water to the nose.

The lungs and trees are thus involved in very similar processes involving similar substances, and it is no surprise then that they have emerged with a similar form. In fact, the lungs are best thought of as an extremely delicate, extremely beautiful gossamer-leaved tree sitting upside down and submerged in a pool of blood!

The blood is gently wafted from the right side of the heart to the left side, at first starting as a river but then resembling more of a delta. It starts at the pulmonary artery and then it branches incessantly until its tributaries are no wider than a single red cell.

At this point they surround the alveoli leaves, and the process of cleaning and re-energising the blood is done. Carbolic acid bubbles up as carbon dioxide and is expelled. The haemoglobin molecules greedily grab oxygen. The blood turns from blue to red and becomes energised.

The delta then starts re-forming into a river again. The capillaries merge and form into veins, veins form into the pulmonary vein and then this drains into the left side of the heart.

Yin

The lungs are therefore almost more blood than they are lung. Imagine a tree standing in all its glory in mid-summer. The space between the leaves, between the branches, needs to be there for the air and light to circulate. Without this space the tree would suffocate. It is the same with the lungs, but the space around the lungs is not just taken by air, it is taken by blood.

This nature of the lungs, whereby they consist of an extremely thin membrane suspended in blood, is why they are considered to be the 'delicate organ' in Chinese medicine. Again, this is similar to leaves on a tree. They are easily damaged by dryness (a process that causes emphysema) because it burns these membranes. Fluid easily fills these spaces as well, because they are an actual space in the body, rather than a potential space.

Just like a tree, the lungs allow connection of our earthly nature to something ephemeral. In the case of a tree it connects sunlight and air to the elements of the earth. The tree allows the trace minerals within the body of our world to be combined with the energy of the sun and building blocks of carbon to create a dazzling world of green. Sunlight and air is not enough to build anything, it is too ephemeral. It needs substance and that substance is provided from the Earth. Once combined it is capable of all the wonders of life.

The sunlight that drives this process equates to the spiritual aspect of our life. As every Englishman knows, sunlight is impermanent, it disappears as quickly as it appears, it cannot be grasped and can only be measured in its intensity. Sunlight is to trees what spirit is to our lungs, but ultimately not in any way that can be 'proven' – it just is. Sometimes in life things have to be accepted as just-so without 'proof'.

What proof there is exists in the innate truth of the assertion. Life is important, despite science telling us that we are just some organic blips on a planet with a timescale that makes us barely a nanosecond in its day. Music is beautiful despite it just being a mathematical representation of acoustic waves. Art means something even though unfeeling machines can create it. Like the trees and their relationship with sunshine, the lungs enable our connection to the ephemeral higher aspects of existence, our God-like quality, despite no objective proof that I am able to offer up.

Of course there is 'proof', but it is subjective proof. Take a few lessons in meditation and notice how the calming of breath takes you to a place that almost exists beyond your body. Conversely, hyperventilate for a while and notice how it leaves you feeling trapped and panicky. These feelings are beyond physics; they are metaphysical and hence more, not less, real than physics. Physical laws are always being proven wrong – Newton's laws trumped Aristotle, Einstein trumped Newton and in times to come Einstein will be proven to have not quite got it right... Science is always being refined, an admission that, in essence, the scientific description of the world isn't quite right.

Yet inner space is a place that we can only discover by ourselves and is therefore innately true, however we experience it. In many philosophical models the only true reality is the reality that is experienced internally, giving birth to Descartes' famous proclamation: 'I think therefore I am.'

Almost all traditions of exploring inner space use either breath or drugs to achieve this, and the drugs are often taken through the lungs!

Yin

Lungs and Blood

The lungs not only regulate the entry of the ephemeral – oxygen and spirit – into our bodies, they also regulate the movement of blood in our chest. Sitting as they do, as an upside-down tree in a river of blood, they exert enormous control over this blood.

Every time we breathe the pressure in our chest changes. When we breathe in, the pressure needs to drop in order for air to be sucked in. This drop in pressure not only sucks in air, it also sucks in blood from the heart. The change in the amount of blood in the heart actually slows it down a little: since the heart takes longer to fill, it takes longer to beat.

Yin   When you breathe out, the reverse happens. The pressure in the chest goes up to expel your breath, blood is forced out of the lungs into the heart and the heart fills more quickly, resulting in the heart beating faster.

In energising the blood with oxygen, the lungs also quantitatively change the nature of the blood. Not only do they transfer carbolic acid for oxygen, but this process also acts to clean up the blood. Acidic blood damages the structure of the red cells, the acid combines with proteins and the cell walls and deforms them. This destruction makes the cells less flexible, and flexibility is one of the most important aspects of red cells. In extremis this acid causes the proteins that form enzymes to unravel and stop working. This aspect of cleaning the blood links the Lung with its paired TaiYin organ – the Spleen. It is an example of what the Chinese describe as transforming 'Dampness' (see page 189). The Lungs squeeze out Dampness through their action of releasing toxins; in this case the specific toxin is carbolic acid. The body stores most of the CO_2 in the blood in this form and it consequently has an osmotic effect, dragging in fluid. By releasing the carbon dioxide the lungs also release water at the same time.

However, especially from a Western perspective, the most important way in which the lungs regulate the blood in the chest is how they filter it.

After every single beat of the heart all the blood from the right side of the heart goes through the lungs to the left side of the heart. The lungs are unique in this way. No other organ receives all the cardiac output. The left-hand side pumps blood to the rest of the organs, but they each receive only a proportion of this. Not only do the lungs receive all the blood from every beat but this is venous blood, stagnant and slow, blood that is liable to have started to clot.

The lungs then have an opportunity to clean this blood, not only of acid and carbon dioxide but also of clots and bubbles that may have formed. It is much better that this occurs in the lungs, since like a delta of a river there is plenty of collateral flow that means that a small clot that becomes lodged is unlikely to cause a problem. Compare this with blood flow into the brain, kidney or even the coronary arteries from the left side of the heart, where a clot would form an 'attack' of some form.[*]

Yin

Obviously there are limits as to what size clots the lungs can deal with. Large clots, which block pulmonary arteries, will cause breathlessness and are known as pulmonary emboli.

This action of the lungs on blood intimately links the lungs to the heart. In Chinese medicine the Heart is seen as the Emperor, the Supreme Controller, and the Lungs are seen as its Minister. The Minister acts to protect the Emperor and regulate his actions. An Emperor that is out of control will ravage his empire and lead to its destruction. The Minister's job is to protect the Emperor from himself and to filter what he receives from his subjects. Breath has this ability to control the mind. Taking slow deep breaths is often the prescription from people concerned about a person's temper: they are exhorting your Emperor to listen to its ministers.

Arm TaiYin – The Lung channel

Your lungs, believe it or not, are actually from the same place as your gut. The reason your mouth and nose join into the same space and then branch off again at the voice box is because they come from the same embryological place. The lung grows out of your primitive gut at a place where your voice box will end up.

Embryologists believe that the lungs and gut emerged from this same place because of feeding. Many fish will filter particles of

---

[*] In this way the lung is behaving as (what the Chinese call) the Pericardium, and protecting the body from causing an 'attack' of (what the Chinese call) Wind. This is why the Chinese call strokes attacks of Wind-Phlegm.

When the lungs grow into the chest, what separates them from the heart is connective tissue. This connective tissue forms the fascia of the chest – pleura and pericardium – but also the membrane between lung and heart. The connective tissue is called the basement membrane and is extremely strong. In this way it catches clots and prevents them from getting to the left side and causing an 'attack'.

Yin   food from the water that goes over their gills. The gills need to be irrigated to ensure the fish has enough oxygen in its blood – clever fish realised you could have a feed at the same time! The place where this interaction occurs in fish is what constitutes the larynx (voice box) in humans.

This all grows out of the Yolk Sac.

The lungs are also unique in that once they start growing they will carry on growing on their own. You can remove the early lung bud and it will keep dividing and growing oblivious to its detachment from the rest of the body.[1] This is not the case with other organs and is emblematic of the fact that the lungs have only one connection to the rest of the body – via the voice box.

Most organs require constant *induction* from other parts of the body – not the lungs. This is very important when we consider the lung channel.

Although the lungs are intimately associated with the blood from the heart, there is a strong fascial barrier between them both, which prevents blood and air mixing – the Blood–Air Barrier.

The Qi connection with the voice box is one reason why, in so much of Chinese medicine, the state of the voice is intimately linked to the quality of Lung Qi. The reason why people who have had a bereavement or loss have a change in the quality and quantity of their voice is because of this connection.

Grief affects our lungs because grief is about loss. Whilst our lungs delicately hold on to the spiritual aspect of our existence, loss reminds us of the impermanence of our lives and the lungs struggle to cope with this.

Despite the fact that the lungs are intimately associated with the blood vessels in the chest, their facial connection exists primarily through the connection with the voice box. This is where the channel gets interesting, for somehow the Lung channel ends up in the arm, and in order to understand how it does that we need to look not at 2000-year-old 'scriptures' but to the 21st century and the world of robotic surgery.

The throat is an extremely complex, and rather scary, part of the body…especially to operate on. Not only do you have the windpipe (vital), carotid arteries (vital), gullet (nice to have), vagal nerve (pretty important) and voice box (useful), but there are also a couple of rather important glands – the thyroid and parathyroid glands.

The thyroid glands are like a metabolic thermostat: turn them up and all the cells in your body work faster, you feel warmer and have more energy. Too fast and you become manic, your eyes bulge and your hair starts falling out. Too slow and you never want to get out of bed. The parathyroid are tiny glands that are buried deep inside this and do some other important stuff (they must do – they're from neural crest cells).

If there is any part of the body where surgeons want to respect the fascial planes it is in the neck! Carotid arteries and jugular veins are not to be trifled with. Surgeons traditionally cut through the skin to get to the thyroid, but despite the proximity of gland to skin (you can even see it when you swallow) this involves cutting across lots of fascial planes. Surgeons do not like cutting through fascial planes; it's when things go wrong.

You see, all good surgeons respect fascial planes, and this is just as true for robot surgeons. The difference is, a robot surgeon isn't restricted by the length of their fingers. A robot surgeon can move along a fascial plane even if that plane starts near the armpit and ends at the throat.

And this is exactly how robot thyroid surgery is done. The incision made for robot thyroid surgery is not made in the throat, it is made at a place near the armpit almost exactly where ancient Chinese medicine designated the 'start' of the Lung channel:[2] underneath the pectoral fascia.

The robot opens a little hole here and then moves along underneath until it arrives at its own little *cave* – the *precervical* fascia. (The Chinese called Acupuncture points 'caves'.)

This technique, while appearing to be more trouble, is actually easier since once you've got into the space under the armpit you don't have to cut through any more fascial planes to get to the thyroid! This is better for the patient because it is a cleaner operation. Patients heal faster, have less bleeding, and

Yin get less damage to their parathyroid glands. Robot surgery has revolutionised how thyroid surgery is done, and will soon become the gold standard.

The robot may be getting in to operate on the thyroid, but the pre-cervical fascia that surrounds this also encases the larynx, the beginning of the Lung channel. The larynx and thyroid are so closely associated that the clinical test to see whether a lump in the neck is in the thyroid is to swallow and see if the lump moves. They even grow out in the same way.

The thyroid gland itself is also related to inspiration and the Lungs. Not only do the hormones released from this gland directly affect your breathing rate but people who lack thyroxine really do seem to lack *inspiration*. In the same way that the adrenal gland is related to the kidney, the thyroid gland may well be the hormonal aspect of the Lungs, a way in which it communicates with the rest of the body. The thyroid gland even grows out in the same way, into the same space and at the same time as the lung; behaving like a *bonsai* lung!

In fact, whilst the lungs govern the *macro*-respiration – the movement of air in and out of our body – the thyroid hormone governs *micro-* or cellular respiration. Cellular respiration is a medical term to describe how quickly the cells burn sugar and oxygen together in the mitochondria. So, in other words, not only does the thyroid gland look like a bonsai lung, it behaves like one too, governing how quickly the little cells 'breathe'.

Thyroid hormones not only behave like the lung does, they are also vitally important in making sure the lung develops fully.[3]

If you look at the description of the Lung channel (for instance, in Peter Deadman's book[4]) it shows a channel that goes from Lung to Adam's apple, and then travels down underneath the clavicle to the armpit (specifically the gap between the clavicular and sternal head of the pectoral muscle). Here it emerges at *Zhong Fu* (The Palace of Gifts) LU-1.

Yin

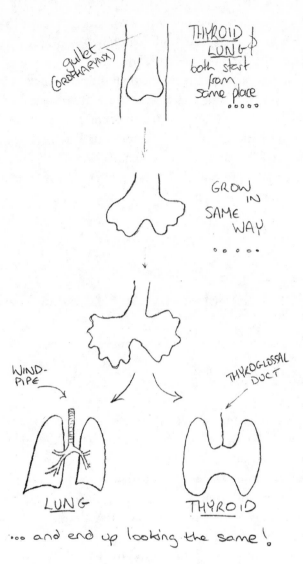

gullet
(OROPHARYNX)

THYROID ↑
LUNG ↓
both start
from
same place
o o o o o

GROW
IN
SAME
WAY
o o o o o

WIND-
PIPE

THYROGLOSSAL
DUCT

LUNG   THYROID

...o and end up looking the same!

What is incredible is that 2000-year-old texts were perfectly describing fascial planes that we are only really understanding with cutting edge robotic surgeons!

The Lung Qi has to go up, because the lung only has one connection to the rest of the body and that is at the voice box. That is why the lung will carry on growing on its own – because its Qi connects at the voice box.

Yin

The Qi flows up from leaves to twigs, twigs to branches, branches to trunk. At the trunk (windpipe) it meets the voice box and here finally it is released. It follows the principles of Qi physics and seeks the external, that is, the fingers. It also flows to the nose, which is why the Lung channel can be used for nosebleeds.

Why does it not flow down at this point to the abdomen?

This is basic Qi physics (explored in Part I). Lung Qi will interact with its paired channel – the Spleen – but it will flow up as this is under pressure. This is no different to a mountain spring where natural laws suggest that the water should continue down, yet the pressure in the system means instead that it bubbles up.

Emergency case reports

The connection with the lung and nose is intuitively obvious and also anatomically real. The nose is part of the long tube that is the gut, and the fascia that encases it extends downwards into the voice box.

This connection between lung and nose means that the Lung channel can be used for nosebleeds and I have used this a number of times, once at my house when a neighbour was insistent that she was not going to have 'that barbaric treatment' of having her nose packed, and many times in the Emergency Department. On numerous occasions the results were dramatic – it was like turning a tap off. The first time I misinterpreted the text in the great Dr Wang Ju Yi's textbook and used *Chi Ze* (Cubital Marsh) LU-5 instead of *Tian Fu* (Celestial Palace) LU-3. I still palpated the channel, though, and found a slippery nodule in the elbow indicating Phlegm. Both neighbours (the patient and her neighbour who had brought her) watched in amazement as the nosebleed stopped within seconds of massaging the point. Afterwards she asked if I thought the Acupuncture had worked!

The point used in the ED the second time was interesting *Yin* because it is rarely used, *Tian Fu* LU-3. It is found on the side of the arm between the insertion of the deltoid muscle and biceps and if you bring your nose to your arm is the point where the two meet. In nosebleeds it is often tender and massage here and along the channel can stop it. Again, the patient was hosing out of the left nostril and the junior doctor who had brought the patient to my attention was keen to practise his nose-packing skills. He was a little put out when I stopped it with massage, but the patient was very impressed. Once again it was like turning off a tap, although on this occasion I needed to massage for a good 5–10 minutes as it would restart again when massage stopped.

From a Western perspective there is obviously no clear reason why a point between the deltoid muscle and the brachialis muscle will stop a nosebleed, but that is before you consider the fascial planes and 3000 years of medical teachings.

The other point that is very useful is *Kong Zui* (Collection Hole) LU-6. This point also translates as 'The Biggest Hole', making it sound like a reality TV programme about…who knows. The point is extremely useful for acute breathlessness, because it is a *cleft* point, a narrowing in the channel where Qi gets stuck. Using this point is like opening this narrowing to allow the Qi through. I have used it on a number of times and it is especially good when the problem is only in the lungs.

People sometimes ask whether/tell me that Acupuncture is psychosomatic and so sometimes I recount the tale of the lady who came in with worsening asthma. The nurse was already fetching the ventolin and steroids, but without the patient even being aware of it I was massaging this point. By the time the ventolin arrived – a few minutes – her asthma had completely resolved. The patient wasn't even aware that me massaging her arm constituted a treatment. (For those with an interest in asthma, her peak flow pre-massage was 320 and post-massage was 550.) I use this as an illustration of how Acupuncture/pressure can work without the patient even being aware it is being done.

Yin   # The Odd Organ

The spleen is the odd organ, which conveniently makes remembering its features easier. Medical students remember it as being 1 inch by 3 inches by 5 inches, weighing 7 pounds, and sitting under the 9th till 11th ribs.

It is not just the numbers of this organ that are odd, though; it also behaves a little oddly.

According to Western medicine it has very little to do with digestion and yet:

- it grows out of the gastrointestinal tract

- it draws its blood supply from the same root as the digestive organs, and

- it is the only organ whose blood drains into the liver that isn't involved in digestion.

The spleen is also odd because it is the only solid organ that can quite happily be removed without any obvious immediate harm to the person. People who rupture their spleen will often have to have it removed, but despite being injurious to a patient's health it is never directly fatal.

(Studies looking at the long-term effects on these patients show surprisingly little effect, save a preponderance to infections from certain bugs and lasting lethargy. However, it is possible other effects are present that simply have never been looked for: for instance, two recent studies – in 2010 and 2012 – showed that these patients have a higher risk of blood clots, thick blood[5] and diabetes.[6])

The oddness of this organ goes on, though, because it is also the only organ that can completely regenerate itself after being removed![7]

What makes it disturbingly odd is that Chinese medicine gives it roles that no sane doctor would ever countenance:

'The ability to think clearly emanates from the Spleen' (*NeiJing SuWen*)

'The Spleen holds the Blood in the Vessels' (*NanJing*)

'The Spleen governs transformation and transportation' (every source on the Spleen!)

…and so on.

Western medicine is far more pragmatic: there are no fancy roles for this organ. It sees the organ as responsible for simply cleaning the cells of the blood. The spleen filters both the red and the white portion of the blood, eliminating the old red cells, acting as a control centre for the white cells and destroying some bacteria in the process. (Very importantly for its Chinese roles, it also both stores platelets and removes old ones from circulation.)

The spleen's micro-architecture is like a fine mesh, and as the red cells pass through this, the old and defective are filtered out. It manages this because, just like people, old red cells become wrinkly, dried out and brittle. Their cell walls become incapable of flexing and bending and the cell becomes stuck in the mesh. White cells in the spleen then break the cell down and recycle the content. Haemoglobin contains vital iron and so is sent onwards to the liver where it is turned into bile, and the rest of the cell is used for bits and bobs (nothing is wasted in the body).

Normal red cells are a biconcave disc – like a doughnut with the middle bit still in. This makes the cells elastic so they can squeeze through narrow gaps: just like Homer Simpson's midriff, the doughnut can flex!

In some people there is a congenital weakness in the red cells that eliminates this flex. In sickle cell disease, abnormal haemoglobin protects against malaria but also causes the cell to deform under stress, making the cell resemble a sickle or spear shape. These get stuck in capillaries. Patients with *spherocytosis* have red cells that resemble a sphere because proteins that are integral to pulling the cell into a doughnut shape are missing. Instead of a disc the cells are spheres and prone to bursting. These too get stuck.

Yin

Yin

Regardless of the cause, all these red cells share an abnormal shape that the spleen is designed to eliminate. In disease, the sheer volume of these abnormal cells then starts to overwhelm the spleen and the spleen gets clogged up and enlarges to try to deal with this extra work. With the constant destruction of red cells it sends the patient anaemic, as the bone marrow cannot make enough new blood. Furthermore, the recycled haemoglobin to the liver becomes excessive and the liver too becomes overwhelmed, causing the patient to become yellow from jaundice.

The spleen is very important for cleaning out tired and defective red cells, and in these cases it is doing its job properly; it is just that the red cells themselves are defective. If the spleen did not clean them out they would clog up the rest of the body and cause serious harm.

In this way the spleen acts as a quality control centre for red cells.

The spleen also has an important role as a centre for immunity. As the blood is passing through the spleen it also passes through a mass of white cells – known as white pulp. These white cells filter and detect bacteria, especially bacteria that have a thick cell wall that makes them resistant to attack – encapsulated bacteria.

Modern armies are based around the same organisation that the body uses to fight infection and enforce order, and in army parlance the spleen is the equivalent of a barracks and command post rolled into one.

Defeated enemies brought here to be interrogated by B-cells have their weaknesses unpicked. Once the enemy's weakness is identified, the B-cells manufacture the equivalent of ballistics, heat-seeking missiles, a chemical that precisely locks on to the enemy called an antibody. From here the army becomes somewhat sci-fi: the B-cells then clone themselves so that they can flood the blood with the precise antibody to defeat the enemy. Once the antibody has locked on to the enemy it acts like a flare, enabling the infantry to see the enemy and attack.

The immune system is a fairly messy and horrible place for invading bacteria. The end point of the immune system involves burning the enemy with hydrogen peroxide, cutting open their skin and then eating them alive. You could almost feel sorry for the bacteria…

Yin

There are other areas of the body that also fulfil the role of command post and barracks – the lymph nodes, thymus and bone marrow – but the spleen also physically traps certain bacteria that are circulating in the blood. The lymph nodes primarily operate in the fascia and this is why splenectomy (removal of the spleen) predisposes to these infections in the blood. These bacteria all share the characteristic of having a thick outer wall, the equivalent of armour plating, which makes them difficult for the immune system to fight.

In the same way that the spleen traps defective red cells it also filters out these fat bacteria: once trapped in the spleen these bacteria become easy prey for the foot soldiers of the immune system – the macrophages (Latin: *macro-* meaning 'big', *-phage* meaning 'eaters').

People who have lost their spleen have impaired ability to fight these organisms and are at risk of pneumonia and meningitis, which is why they are put on lifelong antibiotics.

The last cells in the blood are the platelets. These are tiny little fragments of cells, all originally coming from a giant cell called a megaplatelet, which shatters into tiny pieces like glass. Platelets are vital in clotting, and many drugs that prevent clotting work on platelets.

The spleen destroys old platelets, and diseases of platelets can overwhelm the spleen. The spleen is the most important organ in the body for platelets (after being produced in the bone marrow).

The physical spleen is really two organs in one: an immune command centre and barracks that stores and controls the cells of the immune system; and a quality control centre for red cells and platelets, removing defective ones and recycling their contents. If the Western spleen can be summed up in one word, then, it is blood.

It is difficult to reconcile this vision of the spleen with the Chinese description. The main role for the Chinese Spleen is in:

Yin   Governing transformation and transportation of food into Blood and Qi.

In other words:

Digestion.

Problems with the Spleen treated by Chinese doctors invariably involve digestive complaints – diarrhoea, constipation, poor appetite, abdominal bloating, lethargy and nausea. To be fair, the Chinese consider the Spleen to have an equally important role in creating Blood, but more from absorbing the goodness in the food.

In order to reconcile these two views we have to introduce the pancreas into the picture. And to really confuse things, let's talk about Ming Men!

12 inches of power

'The Kidney on the Right is Ming Men, the Gate of Vitality.' (*NanJing*, Chapter 36, 1st century AD)

Ming Men is the most mysterious force in Chinese medicine. It is talked about as:

'the gate of vitality' (*NanJing*)

'the house of Shen and Jing' (*Contemplations on Unexplored Medical Topics*, c.1584)

'the gorge of mystery, the root of heaven and earth' (*Anthology of Central Harmony*, c.1200)

'the master of the 12 channels, the spark of transformation' (*A Secret Manual from the Stone Chamber*, c.1690)

The strangest thing about Ming Men is that it is always found on the right, never the left. The classics are very particular about that:

'There are two Kidney parts. Actually, not both of them are   *Yin*
Kidneys. The left one is the Kidney, the right one is *Ming*
Men.' (*NanJing*)

Which brings us back to the illustration at the beginning of Part
III (page 122).

The compartment model of the abdomen is a mainstay of
surgical theory and practice. Those precise anatomical dissections
placed the major organs into three compartments, or areas, in the
body: retroperitoneal, anterior pararenal and peritoneal. We call
them ShaoYin, TaiYin and JueYin. These three compartments
do not intermix. This is one of the central tenets of the model:
compartments that intermix can spread infection.

Then someone invented a CT scanner, then someone else
invented the *endoscopic retrograde cholangiopancreatography*.
Seriously, they called it that, or ERCP for short. It's a way of having
a look though your mouth, at your pancreas or liver, and it goes
via the *duodenum*.

If you put these two together you can see whether the person
doing your ERCP has accidentally perforated your duodenum
(lawyers love to find this out).

The radiologists who sit in dark rooms and have a lot of time
to pontificate on the more abstract details of life noticed that
sometimes gas goes into the right kidney space. Not the left, just
the right. So they did a study on it, and found that, indeed, the
second part of the duodenum has very fine connections to the
right kidney.[8]

How strange. This shouldn't happen; according to the
compartment model, the body divides things up to *stop* things
spreading.

The model didn't get it *quite* right: the fascial planes are not
just there to prevent infection (that's a beneficial side-effect), they
are there to guide growth. Which is quite incredible because the
level of control going on here is epic – this really is the Piccadilly
Circus of the body. The *12 inches of power* that constitute this site
of organised chaos.

Yin

This spot is known and loved by anatomists and feared by surgeons. It is the site of the *duodenum digitorum* (Latin: *duodenum* meaning '12', *digitorum* meaning 'fingers' or 'inches'), the 12 inches that everyone needs in order to have a gate full of vitality!

There are 30 or so feet of bowel but the anatomists decided to give this 12 inches its own name. Not only that, but to get more precision they divide it into three-inch segments!

These fine connections from kidney to duodenum are transmitting neural crest cells,[9] Jing made into Qi, which floods into the cavity and causes complete mayhem. In 12 inches of bowel it causes the entire liver, spleen and pancreas to spout out, it makes the duodenum turn right back on itself, it forms all the blood vessels to supply them, and then hangs it all with the *invisible ligament* – the Ligament of Treitz.

The duodenum takes your food, mixes it with Liver Yin (bile) and Spleen Yang (amylase, etc.) and combines it precisely so that when it comes out at the end it is a perfect broth ready to be absorbed. It's like the most ingenious blender ever invented.

The invisible ligament is at the end where it comes out. This ligament is so faint that it cannot be seen on even the best scans – only dissection will reveal it. It holds up the last part of the duodenum like a collar-and-cuff type sling holding an arm, and decides how quickly food will go into the rest of the bowel. At its other end it wraps tightly around the aorta (heart) and inserts into the vertebra of the back.

This invisible ligament is why the Chinese have a connection between Small Intestine and Heart.

Spleen Yang – The Pancreas

The broth that comes out under the direction of the invisible ligament is a product of all these interactions, but it is the alkaline fire of the pancreas that charges it. The pancreas is ignored by Chinese medicine…and that is just bizarre.

There can be no doubting its existence, but the only reference that is made to it is in the *NanJing*, with regard to the 'greasy organ' that is the site of…*Ming Men*.

The pancreas isn't Ming Men, though – Ming Men is the Jing/ neural crest cells that lies here, that enables the great organisation.

The pancreas and spleen are really one organ. They look as shown in the illustration.

Yin

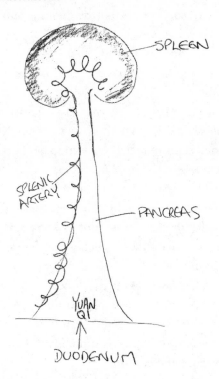

The pancreas and spleen organs grow out from the duodenum. The pancreas starts first and then the spleen organ caps it off. The pancreas sits in the pararenal space (TaiYin), but at its tip it becomes intraperitoneal (JueYin) and it does this by tucking into the fascia of the spleen.

It looks like a volcanic explosion and in a way it is. Ming Men has boiled the Blood in the ShaoYin channel and caused an enormous volcanic eruption of TaiYin. At its apex this forms a mushroom cloud which forces its way into the JueYin.

Yin   The pancreas and spleen are so closely linked that they could be considered one organ. Embryologically the pancreas requires signals from the spleen to form.[10] They share arterial blood supply – the splenic artery – and also drain into the same vein. The reason splenectomy is thought to make diabetes worse is because the spleen even contains stem cells for the pancreas.[6]

Furthermore, the spleen is the only solid organ that can regenerate. The reason for this may be that it is only half the organ that has been taken!

If any further proof is needed, then it is that extra spleens are sometimes found within the pancreas, for this is the line which it grows out from![11]

Linking spleen and pancreas is not just a matter of convenience; there is strong evidence that these two organs share common beginning, blood supply, fascial connection, and even support each other in adult life.

In Chinese medicine they are Spleen Yin and Spleen Yang. They are the Yin and Yang of digestion. As we shall see, whilst the pancreas provides the Digestive Fire to cook and transform the food, the spleen regulates how quickly that happens through the hormone serotonin.

Calling the Chinese organ the Spleen is thus confusing: it should be the Spleen–Pancreas or Spancreas. A name may just be a name, but the Chinese medical community is using a name that means something completely different. When they talk about Spleen, they mean pancreas too!

We have to change the name of this channel now, and after much deliberation I have come up with…

I've no idea…

…but I think the pancreas is definitely Spleen Yang so that's what I'm going to call it.

The pancreas has two functions. One of these is to provide the enzymes, the Digestive *Fire*, to break down food into smaller bits: this is the *transformation* of food. Without this fire, food would be excreted in a similar state to how it entered.

The other function is to provide the hormone (insulin) to allow   *Yin*
the *transportation* of this food (sugar). Diabetes is the disease where
the pancreas fails to produce enough insulin. Medics know it as
starving in the midst of plenty: whilst there is plenty of sugar in the
blood, the cells cannot take it up without the insulin. The insulin
enables this transportation of food.

The Chinese Spleen function of transformation and
transportation mirrors the functions of the pancreas perfectly.

One of the most important hormones for regulating both these
processes, but especially insulin release, is serotonin. Serotonin has
a peculiar, nay, *odd* role in this process. Normally serotonin would
act as a simple on/off trigger like most hormones, but in insulin
secretion – a critical function in our bodies – serotonin really
appears to *regulate* this process.[12]

You could probably find roles for all the hormones with
insulin, so important is it in the body: serotonin and insulin are so
intimate, however, that cell biologists will monitor insulin release
by measuring serotonin release![12]

This hormone provides the connection between spleen, Spleen,
and pancreas.

Spleen (Yang) transforms Dampness

Dampness is a condition of the body where there is too much fluid.

There's no doubt that fluid can accumulate in the body, as both
heart and kidney failure are treated with diuretics to eliminate this.
While both East and West agree that there is a dampness that can
arise from pump failure (heart), or failure to drain fluid (kidney),
there is another type of Dampness that the West ignores but is
endemic in many diseases such as irritable bowel syndrome (IBS).

This Dampness is caused by Spleen Yang (pancreas) deficiency
and is different in nature to heart or kidney failure: Spleen Yang
(pancreas) Dampness is a Dampness of impaired metabolism
rather than an inability to move fluids.

Yin

Spleen Yang-type Dampness presents differently to heart and kidney overload. In heart and kidney failure the Dampness falls down and creates swelling in the ankles. Spleen Yang Dampness results in fluid accumulating around the midline, beer bellies and abdominal bloating being examples of this. The complexion is often very different too: heart and kidney failure often result in a grey, dusky or blue complexion; patients with Spleen Yang Dampness look yellow.

In fact, the term 'sallow complexion' describes Spleen Yang deficiency almost perfectly.

People who have overactive spleens do go yellow. The word jaundice comes from the French for yellow – *jaune* – and the term jaundice is used to describe the yellowness of the skin. This jaundice is created by excess bilirubin, caused by the breakdown of defective red cells. The yellowness of the Dampness in Spleen Yang deficiency is different to the bright yellow of spleen excess seen in blood diseases.

The division of diseases into those of excess and deficiency is one of the central tenets of Chinese medicine: excess conditions are caused by something extra added to the body – typically a pathogen or in this case bilirubin – whereas deficiency is caused by the body not having enough to do its job properly.

By their nature, excess conditions are more dramatic and obvious; deficiency conditions mean that something is lacking. The picture is, however, normally mixed.

Patients with jaundice often become so yellow that it would be comical if not so tragic, whereas the sallowness created by pancreas deficiency is subtle. These are people who do not have an overactive spleen creating excess bilirubin, but instead an underactive pancreas allowing accumulation of toxins and hence fluid.

One of the commonest groups to see this condition in is people with irritable bowel syndrome. IBS is a name for a wide range of gastrointestinal symptoms and it is a *diagnosis of exclusion*. If the doctor finds nothing wrong in his tests then your gastrointestinal symptoms are thrown in the bin that is 'IBS'.

No wonder it is so poorly managed and generally ignored by Western doctors – it isn't even really a diagnosis. However, Chinese medicine has very clear ideas about what is going on and at its heart it is often the simple result of a deficient pancreas allowing Dampness to develop.

In the case of pancreas-deficiency Dampness it emerges not, as in kidney or heart failure, as a result of failure to eliminate fluids, but as a result of osmosis. In other words, the Dampness appears first as toxic metabolites, which then drag water in behind them.

This process, the way in which water follows dissolved substances, is called osmosis and is critical in normal functioning of all organisms. Our cells use it to balance the quantity of fluid within the cells and also outside of the cells.

When metabolites appear that shouldn't be there (toxins) this upsets the balance (homeostasis). The toxins attract water to them and, since the body is unable to deal with them efficiently, both the water and toxins linger. This is what the Chinese call Dampness and it is no surprise that it is found most commonly in the gut, since the gut's composting nature is extremely prone to brewing… 'toxins'.

Dampness becomes self-perpetuating: it tends to make things sluggish and this process reduces the ability to clear things from the system. The result of this stagnation is that metabolism slows and toxins are more likely to be formed.

Many medics dislike this term *toxins*, but toxins are simply any substances that are present in higher concentrations than normal, or not healthy to cellular function. To pretend that there are no toxins in our body is disingenuous.

An example of a toxin is excess sugar, caused when the pancreas fails to make enough insulin. In normal concentration sugar is vital to the functioning of every cell, but in diabetes levels of sugar rise and instead of becoming healthy it becomes toxic. Once the levels get high enough, the sugar overflows through the kidneys, sucking water with it through osmosis. As a result the patient starts to constantly pee, but is always thirsty trying to replenish the lost

Yin

Yin fluids. Eventually the patient becomes severely dehydrated and only insulin can save them.

Even though the above example causes massive dehydration, and therefore would appear to be an example of dryness, it is driven by an osmotic Dampness created by excess sugar. The sugar and water combined overflow and pour out of the body, leaving the contents within sweeter, stickier and altogether nastier.

This is an example of what time does to Dampness. It turns it into something more pathological, something nastier, something that in Chinese medicine is called Phlegm – congealed Dampness.

Everyone knows what phlegm is – we cough it up when we have a cold. Thanks to medical science we now know that what occurs in the arteries of people with coronary disease is also 'phlegm'. This substance, whilst technically called an *atherosclerotic plaque*, resembles cheese, is sticky, hard and looks like…phlegm. Phlegm can also occur in our bowel motions as mucus, coat the inside of our arteries supplying our organs and silt up the inner workings of our organs.

There is even a kidney condition where it creates 'casts', which are perfect phlegmy miniature casts of the inside of the kidney (see, I told you I learnt something as the last ever renal houseman).

Phlegm is Dampness that has been worked on by Heat. Dampness in the body is not inert: the body is naturally a warm place and so it alters Dampness in the same way that a low flame will act on a broth. It will thicken it and concentrate it; and thicken it more until it resembles not a liquid but a sticky paste. Depending on what the initial constituents of the broth were, the paste will have different properties and appearances, but its characteristics will be the same: it will be sticky, hard and difficult to remove.

'Aaahhhh!' I hear the pathologists say, looking up from their microscopes. 'All those things – the phlegm from colds, the atherosclerotic plaques, the mucus in stools – they are the product not of boiling but of an immune reaction. The "phlegm" is dead white cells and their enemies.'

This is true, of course. Mucus and phlegm, and even atherosclerotic plaques, are chock-a-block with dead white cells…

Yin

But! Why are the white cells there? The white cells are responding to a pathogen or toxin; this pathogen may be bacterial, viral, or even something like asbestos, or toxic cholesterol. The white cells create in-*flame*-ation to deal with it:

$$\text{Dampness} + \text{Heat} = \text{Phlegm}$$

The Phlegm of Chinese medicine can be a lot subtler than these gross examples, though. The pathogens in colds or abscesses are obvious – we get sick from a bug and the connection with the phlegm becomes self-evident. In these cases there is enormous production of Dampness from bacterial or viral toxins and the fever quickly boils this to create a Phlegm whilst the immune system works to keeps it localised.

In the case of atherosclerotic plaques this is subtler still – the process is slow and takes years. The only reason we pay it much attention is because the effects it has on the body are so dramatically devastating. The process of slow phlegm formation can occur anywhere, though. The phlegm occurring elsewhere causes conditions less known to laymen:

- Adhesions in the abdomen: these look like white sticky strands and tie the bowel together causing obstruction.

- Fascitis/tendonitis: this causes pain as a result of increased friction and inability of the tendons to move.

- Sinusitis: chronic phlegm formation in the sinuses.

- Glomerulonephritis: inflammation of the kidneys.

- Bronchitis.

- (Visceral) fat around our organs which is known to be a serious risk factor for illness.

In fact, any organ or tissue can be affected by this substance: it is ubiquitous in its pathogenicity.

This ubiquity can appear to limit its usefulness. Western medicine relies on reductionism to guide its treatments and such a catch-all would appear to limit guided treatment.

Yin

For instance, the exact causes of atherosclerotic plaques are mired in tome upon tome of Western research and this research enables cures and advice, treatments and prognosis. However, when you get to the nitty-gritty of what it involves, it all boils down to a combination of Dampness- and Heat-forming Phlegm.

As an example, risk factors for heart plaques include:

- smoking (Heat- and toxin-forming)

- diabetes (Damp-forming)

- high cholesterol (Phlegm itself)

- family history (predilection towards forming Phlegm)

- obesity (Phlegm)

- poorly expressed anger (this emotion causes Heat).

Splenectomy (removal of the spleen) is also a risk factor[13, 14] because the spleen helps control Dampness.

To a Western doctor a diagnosis of Phlegm is so vague as to be meaningless, but it is all in the interpretation. Diagnosing Phlegm is useful because the treatment always follows the same lines: clear the Phlegm, reduce Dampness and Heat, and strengthen the Organ.

The West follows this same treatment principle. For instance, in a heart attack, Western medicine would open the coronary artery (clear Phlegm), treat the diabetes (reduce Dampness) and advise to stop smoking (reduce Heat).

In Chinese medicine it would involve…rushing to a Western hospital, admitting that sometimes 'their' medicine was better, and pleading for a Western cardiologist to stent the artery, get the insulin for the diabetes…

And then…treating the individual causes of Damp and Heat.

It is worth pointing out at this point that, even though Western medicine now has the best acute treatments for coronary artery disease, the Chinese had described the cause of this 2000 years before Edward Jenner wrote this in his diary in 1783:[15]

Yin

After having examined the more important parts of the heart, without finding anything by means of which I could account either for his sudden death or the symptoms preceding it, I was making a transverse section of the heart pretty near its base, when my knife struck against something so hard and gritty, as to notch it. I well remember looking up to the ceiling, which was old and crumbling, conceiving that some plaster had fallen down. But on further scrutiny the real cause appeared: the coronaries were becoming bony canals.

A quite remarkable note, which lays the foundation for almost all of cardiology.

The Chinese, however, have described for thousands of years – beginning in the *NeiJing SuWen* – a syndrome of 'Chest Obstruction' that led to the patient turning blue and collapsing. They described how this was caused by Blood and Phlegm stagnation in the *collateral vessels* of the Heart.

This is as succinct an explanation of a coronary heart attack as you will get today: if you substitute *coronary* for *collateral*. Maybe Jenner's grasp of Chinese was better than mine, for his other great discovery – vaccinations – had precedence in China way before he was born.[16]

Phlegm, then, is a substance that emerges from Dampness and binds up the tissues of our body. But this chapter is about the pancreas – what has it got to do with the pancreas? Furthermore, when is this all going to tie in with the spleen?

In Western medicine the spleen is absolutely vital in 'cleaning' red blood cells. To be fair, this is done by removing the 'dirty' ones, but the result is the same – it cleans the blood and enables it to move smoothly.

Smooth flow of blood is not as simple as it sounds – because the critical aspect of this smooth flow at the capillary level is the deformability of the cells. Red cells, incredibly, are twice as wide as the capillaries they need to get down, and to do this they need to deform.[17]

That funny biconcave, doughnut shape is no accident: this allows them to be squashed into a sphere and so get through tighter

Yin spots. Red cells that can't flex either get stuck or split. Split red cells are bad news; they may only form the world's smallest bruise but since when are bruises good?

Anyone who has had a bad cough knows that phlegm is sticky, and this applies to the blood too. Phlegm in the blood causes the red cells to become sticky and hence stiff, and as a result they get stuck.

The cause of the sallow complexion that is seen so often in irritable bowel syndrome is a result of this increased stickiness. Sticky or inflexible red cells become stuck and refuse to pass through smoothly, or break and cause inflammation. The area becomes hypoxic and swells, and instead of being able to see the blood we are only able to see the sticky fluid that has replaced it. It is symptomatic of a poor microcirculation – a sallow complexion – and that is why these patients can look anaemic and pale even when the red cell levels are normal.

Fibromyalgia is another disease where the red cells get deformed and stuck,[18] and in Chinese medicine this condition is felt to be due to Blood stagnation often caused by Dampness.

Many doctors don't believe that fibromyalgia even exists, when in fact it is just that Western medicine is barely advanced enough to understand it. What fibromyalgics have is a very gentle form of the same problem that sickle cell anaemics get!

The reason that the ancients Chinese texts state that 'the Spleen abhors Dampness' is because of this relationship between rheology (the study of the flow of blood), Dampness and the Spleen; but this still does not fully explain how the spleen and the pancreas are related.

Extraordinary, bah!

There is a point on the Spleen channel called *Gong Sun* (Grandfather Grandson) SP-4. Through the mists of time it has acquired not one but two names. One of these translates as 'minute connecting vessels'. The point itself is one of the most important and one of the most well-used points in the body for it is also the opening point of what is called the *Chong Mai*.

'Chong' means 'surging' and 'Mai' means 'channel'. The classics say the Chong Mai can be felt in the abdomen as the Surging channel and the similarities between the Chong Mai and what we call the aorta and arterial system are too numerous to ignore. For all intents and purposes they are the same thing.

The Chong Mai is one of the *extraordinary channels*. The ordinary channels exist as real entities that can be dissected out in the fascia, but the extraordinary channels exist as relationships that occur deeper than this. If the channels are like roads that enable movement for cars, the extraordinary channels are like the gravel or tarmac used to make the roads. If the ordinary channels are like rivers running through the body, the extraordinary channels represent the tiny currents of water that run between the grains of the soil and between the roots of plants. If the ordinary channels are like fibre-optic wires carrying thousands of signals in a city, the extraordinary channels are the gossip that occurs between the people in the city.

The extraordinary channels are more primal and more important than the ordinary channels and exist from the moment the first cell divides. When the ordinary channels become blocked, it is the extraordinary channels that ensure movement can still occur.

In fact, it is the ordinary channels that are really extraordinary; these are amazing since there are millions of cells all using the same pathway.

In the case of the Chong Mai, this (extra)ordinary channel is the channel of blood vessels. Blood vessels permeate every part of our being. They bring the life-blood of our existence to our cells. The blood vessels are themselves 'channels', channels that transmit not so much Qi but blood.

It is no coincidence that the 'opening point' on the Chong Mai translates as 'minute connecting vessels'. Excess Dampness in the body creates stickiness and this stickiness in turn restricts movement through the tiniest blood vessels. These tiny blood vessels then become obstructed, the blood supply becomes restricted and the tissues become sallow.

Yin

Yin   The minute connecting vessels that this point is named after are those minute connecting vessels called *capillaries*. These are the smallest of the blood vessels that provide individual cells with nutrients. This point is used because it regulates the spleen function of controlling these, specifically by encouraging the spleen to remove a hormone that closes up the minute connecting vessels.

The Chinese phrase to sum up this relationship is:

The Spleen holds the blood in the Vessels

which is both poetic and precise.

How could the spleen affect the capillaries in this way? To answer this we have to look at a hormone that most people associate with feeling good, legal or otherwise, the hormone of Prozac and Ecstacy – serotonin!

Conveniently (for me) the name serotonin simply means blood vessel (*sero-*) contractor (*-tonin*). So, the link between capillaries closing up and serotonin is a given. How does it relate to the spleen, though?

Serotonin is best known as the feel-good hormone, but what is less known is that over 95 per cent of serotonin is found not in the brain but in the gut! In fact, serotonin should probably have been called *enterotonin* as its Italian discoverer Vittorio Erspamer named it. This was after its ability to make the gut (*entero-*) contract (*-tonin*).

Sadly, neither Erspamer's moniker nor 'serotonin' won out and its official, rather dry, name is 5-hydroxytryptamine (5-HT).

As is now becoming patently obvious in the world of medicine, hormones and neurotransmitters are not only indistinguishable, but have a diverse and ubiquitous role throughout our body. Serotonin is no exception; it is found in gut and blood, brain and heart. The vast amounts of serotonin stored in our gut are vital to moving food through at an appropriate rate. Throughout the gut are tiny glands rich in serotonin; when the gut is disturbed by infection or toxins the storage cells release a surge of serotonin to expel the contents of the gut.

In Western medical circles this surge goes by many names: *Yin*
Delhi Belly, Montezuma's Revenge, Cairo Two-Step. But it all ends
in the same place…if you get there in time.

This surge of serotonin also overflows into our blood where it
overwhelms the ability of platelets to mop it up. It finds its way
to the vomiting centre in our brainstem, where it causes us to
reject and eject the offending contents. The result is known to all
but the luckiest of people as an urgent need to get to the toilet.
The knowledge of serotonin's actions has allowed drug companies
to produce the most successful anti-vomiting drug that we have,
which works by blocking the specific serotonin receptor (5-HT^3)
in the vomiting centre on the floor of the IVth Ventricle in the
brain (not a cool place to hang out).

Even though it is the same chemical – serotonin – it can have
multiple different effects in the body by using different receptors.
They are named, again quite dryly: 5-HT^1, 5-HT^2…all the way
to 5-HT^7.

In this way one hormone produced by a single gland can have a
wide variety of different effects throughout the body. This is similar
to how Chinese medicine teaches that the Spleen keeps blood in
the vessels, allows you to think clearly, creates saliva, and ensures
transformation and transportation.

The serotonin in our brain is not limited to vomiting, however,
but is also integral to what we call *obsessive-compulsive disorder*
(OCD). This condition is considered a brain disorder in Western
medicine but the Chinese have always considered it a problem of
digestion. The sayings to 'ruminate on', to 'digest', to 'chew over'
are all digestive phrases that are equally applicable to thinking;
even the phrase 'to mull over' is from a process whereby drinks are
made more palatable and digestible…

This etymological connection is not coincidence: in Chinese
medicine the Spleen/pancreas is the source of the Qi that enables
us to think clearly. Over-thinking, worry and even excessive study
are processes that adversely affect our guts. The reason why IBS
sufferers appear to be neurotic worriers is because it is another
manifestation of the same disease: the serotonin disturbance that

Yin   is causing their harried bowels is also depleting their ability to think clearly. Their 'neurosis' is often seen as a problem to general practitioners, but it would be more helpful to see it as another symptom of their gut pathology.

OCD is an example of a problem of thinking that presents with repetitive behaviour and worrying. We have all had those moments where we have had to go home to check the gas was not left on, but an obsessive-compulsive can be paralysed by an inability to dispel these thoughts. Some obsessive-compulsives are so worried about germs that they repetitively wash their hands until they bleed.

This syndrome responds fantastically to boosting brain serotonin levels with Prozac and other 5-HT drugs. As the painstakingly accurate and fastidiously researched book *Obsessive Compulsive Disorder Research* states:[19]

> the involvement of the $5\text{-}HT^2$ receptor in OCD is broadly accepted.

In fact, SSRIs (Selective Serotonin Reuptake Inhibitors, the class of drugs of which Prozac is a member) deserve far more credit for successfully treating this than their dubious record with 'depression' (suicide is more common after SSRIs[20]).

The only problem with Prozac in OCD is that the disease often relapses once Prozac is stopped. I hope by this point the reason for this would be obvious.

No?

OK… The disease is not originating in the brain: it is being caused by abnormal serotonin metabolism in the gut!

This abnormal serotonin biochemistry causes the brain to malfunction. Prozac works, for sure, but it is a sticking plaster over the true cause – abnormal (spleen) metabolism of serotonin.

'Ahh, hah!' I hear the physiologists say. 'Perhaps the good doctor has made a mistake!' Serotonin cannot get into the brain, it's barred by the and neurovascular unit (a.k.a. the blood–brain barrier). Only VIPs (Very Important Proteins and stuff) can get in and serotonin is not on the guest list. Sure, it gets onto the floor

of the IVth Ventricle, but this place is also known as the vomit *Yin*
centre – anyone can get in there!

This is all true of course…in health – but what scientists are
finding in disease is that raised serotonin levels can bypass the
barrier between blood and brain and cause havoc with the brain
function.[21] Chronically raised serotonin levels somehow manage
this and cause the very same 5-HT[2] receptors to be activated that
are implicated in OCD.[22]

Serotonin is thus clearly a bowel hormone that affects the
brain, as much as the other way around…

One of the most controversial use of serotonin drugs is in IBS
itself. It is controversial because, almost by definition, IBS will not
kill you whereas the drugs might.[23]

However, the drug companies spent a lot of money
investigating the serotonin–IBS link and came up with two drugs
for treating IBS that they voraciously pushed. The first is a 5-HT[3]
receptor drug which is used when diarrhoea predominates; the
second is a 5-HT[4] receptor drug which is used when constipation
predominates. The merits of both drugs are dubious since,
despite sometimes having positive effects, both are known to
cause fatalities; but the pharmacology is intriguing as it shows the
integral link between serotonin and IBS.

What these drugs illustrate is that serotonin is produced by
the cells in the gut as a guide to what the bowel should be doing.
There is a balance, and the balance needs to be finely tuned. Too
much and you have to rush to the toilet; too little and you spend
your whole day trying to go. Serotonin is like the speed dial on
your bowels.

Dampness in the body emerges as a result of toxins and these
are easily produced in the gut when the composting nature of the
gut goes wrong. Serotonin is the hormone that controls the speed
at which food moves through the gut and so the amount of toxins,
and hence Dampness, that emerges.

While this is all very interesting, it still has not explained what
this has all got to do with the spleen…

Yin   A single piece of research from 1962...

The way in which the Chinese linked over-thinking, the ability to hold blood in the vessels, Dampness, and digestion was born out of years of patient observation and experimentation into the effects of herbs, toxins and Acupuncture points. The Chinese did not necessarily understand that there was a common hormone – serotonin – that linked all these things, but they noticed the connections through observation.

Why did they link all these effects to the spleen, the odd, small, disc-shaped, bloody organ sitting next to the left kidney?

Who knows, but what is remarkable is that the spleen does have a very, very intimate link with serotonin:

- 95 per cent of the serotonin in our body is in the gut.

- 99 per cent of serotonin in the blood is found in platelets: platelets greedily gobble it up when it spills over from the gut.

- The spleen stores and destroys platelets.

In fact, the spleen is the most important organ for platelets in the body: it houses up to a third of the platelets, and removes the abnormal ones from circulation.

When disorders of platelets are present the spleen is invariably involved; in fact, treatment for platelet disorders sometimes involves *removing* the spleen!

If the spleen cleans the blood of platelets, and the platelets clean the blood of serotonin, you would expect the spleen to have high levels of serotonin...

...but the reverse is true.[24]

In fact, this single piece of research,[24] from 1962, in the absence of any contradictory findings, brings us to a remarkable conclusion:

The spleen, it appears, is the number one organ for cleaning serotonin from the blood (via the platelets).

If the spleen is cleaning the blood of serotonin, then it is regulating all the things that serotonin regulates:

Yin

- It is regulating the amount of insulin released to 'transport' food via $5HT^1$ receptors in the pancreas.

- It is regulating serotonin's effects on platelets and clotting via $5HT^2$ and the amount of serotonin that leaks into the brain and causes over-thinking via the same receptor.

- It is regulating the baseline amount of serotonin in the blood around the gut that will either cause diarrhoea ($5HT^3$)…

- …or constipation ($5HT^4$).

- In these ways, with its brother the pancreas, it regulates absorption of food and therefore our ability to form strong muscles and keep good body tone (two other functions of the spleen).

In fact, when you substitute the word 'serotonin' for 'spleen' it does almost everything the Acupuncture textbooks say.

Why then do these things not go completely wrong when the spleen is removed?

Many of them do go partially wrong: the blood becomes thicker and stickier; the patient becomes more prone to toxin build-up and Dampness from increased infections and higher sugar levels; and the patient becomes more tired and lethargic. In the main, though, the patient's life continues on without too much disturbance.

The reason for this is twofold.

First, the spleen is only one half of the Spleen – you still have your pancreas, which probably takes over some of the roles and probably provides the signals for those spleens that regenerate. The two organs are each half of a duality. This is why the spleen has stem cells for the pancreas, and the pancreas has accessory spleens.

Second, some of the functions of the spleen are taken over by the liver. Within a few months the platelet level comes back to normal as the liver takes over the process of eliminating platelets.

Yin With the platelets regulated, the blood levels of serotonin can be normalised and the functions of the Spleen-Yin become regulated.

The liver doesn't do this quite as well, though, which is why diabetes and blood clots become more common.

The spleen is an odd organ, and this ability to be removed and its functions taken over by other organs is *very* odd.

It's a weird organ…

Furthermore, I've cheated a bit; it's not even *technically* in the anterior pararenal space, but its brother is.

Leg TaiYin – The Spleen channel

The space occupied by the pancreas is the anterior pararenal space, which communicates with the oesophagus upwards and hence the lung.

Downwards it flows into the femoral sheath, where the spleen channel starts at SP-12 – *Chong Men*. The name Chong Men has a double meaning. First, because it is found next to the pulsating vessel (in the femoral sheath); and second, because it reflects its influence over the Chong Mai.

The channel somewhat follows the artery down into the leg (see illustration on page 166) but then veers off oddly. I've spent enough time on this weirdo organ; nearly time to move on to the Bodyguard! But first…

Emergency case report

How does the Spleen/Pancreas channel work in practice?

I had one patient who came into the Emergency Department with chronic vaginal bleeding: drip, drip, drip for four weeks.

It was like a tap that couldn't quite shut completely. She looked sallow, weak and seemed needy but her lab work-ups were all normal. In the language of Western medicine she was a heart-sink, not because her physical heart was sinking, but because it could make my heart sink!

She was menopausal and the gynaecologists told me to whack her on some hormones and get her home. Incredibly, at that point my consultants were letting me use needles and, of course, she was more than happy to try.

This is the incredible thing about Acupuncture: when faced with Western medicine at its wishy-washy worst (What's causing my bleeding...? Err...don't know... Take these hormones, though), people are almost always willing to try it. Informed consent is the most wonderful thing ever to have happened to Western medicine – it puts the patient in the driving seat. Not many doctors inform the patient of the risk of a CT scan (1 in 2000 lifetime chance of a fatal cancer), but it can allow the patient to take the informed decision not to have it and save you a lot of arse-covering hassle. Much stuff done in hospitals is done because lawyers' 'retrospectovision' is always 20–20 – a lawyer always seems to know what was going to happen *after* it happened. To be fair, doctors rarely take the time to explain all the risks and benefits, but informed consent puts the patient in the driving seat, not the lawyers *or* the doctors.

This patient gave her informed consent and in this case Chinese medicine had all the answers. She did not have 'peri-menopausal bleeding'; she had a spleen deficiency manifesting in abnormal serotonin metabolism. Her sallow complexion was a result of poor microcirculation, her neediness a serotonin imbalance in her brain, and the drip-drip caused by platelets that couldn't quite do their job because they didn't have enough *tone*.

Needles in *Zu San Li* (Leg Three Mile) ST-36 and *San Yin Jiao* (Three Yin Crossing) SP-6 stopped the bleeding for the first time in four weeks, improved her complexion and actually made her feel better! She left without the hormones, cured, and the hospital saved money.

Yin

JueYin (Returning Yin)

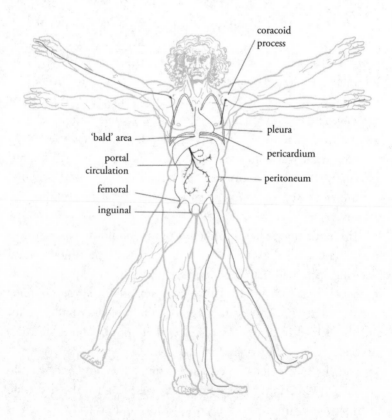

coracoid process

pleura

'bald' area

pericardium

portal circulation

peritoneum

femoral

inguinal

The Emperor's Bodyguard

Yin

The Heart is so important that it needs protection and this protection comes from the Pericardium.

In the ancient philosophy of Chinese medicine, the set-up of society mirrored the internal dynamics of our body (a metaphysical fractal). The *NeiJing SuWen* talks about the Heart being the Emperor and an Emperor needs guards and a palace. If anyone could freely access the Emperor then he would be vulnerable to not only physical attack but also mental and emotional attack. The trials and tribulations of all his subjects could overwhelm him, and so it is the court's job to ensure that what reaches him is appropriate.

The Heart not only provides the beating pulse of life, but as explained before it also enables our ability to relate at a loving level. It does not govern how we think about these relationships; it leaves this to the brain.

In order to relate, our Heart needs to be open. The process of opening your Heart to somebody, or letting somebody into your Heart, is a process that occurs at an emotional level. People can be 'shut off' from others or 'open hearted', and both of these can be appropriate at different times. The Heart may enable us to relate to others, but to do this properly it needs a gatekeeper, and the gatekeeper is the Pericardium.

The Pericardium grows from a part of the embryo called the *pleuropericardial* folds. These grow inwards from the front of our body, roughly on a line with where our nipples will be. They will separate the abdomen from the chest and they will do this by forming the diaphragm. Above the diaphragm it forms the pericardium and, below it, it directs the growth of the liver. This is the origin of the JueYin channel in Acupuncture.

The pericardium is unique within the body. All organs are wrapped in fascia but, apart from the pericardium, this consists of two layers – one attached to the organ, the other to the body wall.

Yin

These layers serve both a functional purpose in enabling movement and an energetic purpose in channelling Qi and keeping order.

The heart, however, is wrapped in three layers. The first two layers are similar to the fascia that wraps most other organs, thin to the point of transparency, enabling both energetic and physical organ to move. The extra third layer is extremely thick and strong fascia, thousands of times thicker than the first two and grown out from the chest wall. This is the layer unique to the heart and is known as the *fibrous pericardium*.

The function of the fibrous pericardium in Western medicine is a bit boring. It does protect the heart from rupture and from invading pathogens but, like all fascia, is generally ignored. It rarely gets diseased; even the condition known as 'pericarditis' turns out to be a bit of a misnomer, since the pathological hallmarks are more accurately in the epicardium of the heart. People born with pericardial defects do carry a higher risk of heart disease, showing that its role as heart protector is accurate.[1]

The function of protection is similar to the Chinese medicinal function of the Pericardium, except that in Chinese medicine it also prevents entry of pathogenic energy. The Pericardium functions as a gate, allowing loved ones into your Heart but preventing people who might emotionally harm you from entering.

Without this function we could allow our Hearts to become *entangled* with anyone else's Hearts. Some people do allow this: they fall in love easily, maybe inappropriately; treat strangers like loved ones; give away their energy freely. And then get hurt easily.

The phrase 'to wear your heart on your sleeve' is thought to refer to medieval jousting and the tradition of wearing your patron's colours on your arm. However, it could equally refer to someone who was leaving their heart vulnerable for anyone to access.

In extremis, people with open hearts can become manic, do 'crazy' things and give away all their things. As far as Chinese medicine is concerned it is not necessarily a problem that originates in their head, but is instead because their Pericardium is not functioning properly, leaving their Heart too open. It is as though the Emperor's court has disappeared and anyone can walk into his palace, although instead of hiding away he goes and parties with everyone.

Conversely, instead of being too open, access to the Heart can be too closed. Now the Heart struggles to connect with anybody else. The person seems shut off and distant, as though they have no Heart (although it is just not open for business).

Whilst this is all very interesting, is there any way that the Pericardium could actually function like this at a physical level?

> The heart has reasons that reason cannot know. (Blaise Pascal, mathematician)

It is logically impossible to ascertain the working of the *emotional* heart, and yet that is what we are trying to do. To get to these reasons we move to the edges of science where it starts to resemble science fiction rather than science fact…

The fibrous pericardium is a thick matted matrix of collagen fibres. Collagen fibres not only create electricity but also conduct electricity too (fully explored in Part I). This conduction is direction-able so that they act a like a mesh of nano-sized insulated wires. The consequence of this thick matted matrix is that the heart is surrounded by both a physical and an electrical shield.

Each collagen fibre will hold its own electrical charge and create electrical charge each time it is deformed by the beating of the heart: the process of piezo-electricity. In cadavers the fibrous pericardium seems inert and dull, like tough cloth, but in the body it looks shiny and vital, a living liquid crystal of collagen. This crystal will both generate and transmit electrical energy, and in doing so it will create a static electrical field which is capable of interacting, modifying or even blocking other electrical fields.

This latter point is not entirely fanciful. In Western medicine we do use crude energy medicine, and we use it on the heart. Electromagnetic shocks to help the heart are known as *defibrillation* and can be used to change its rhythm.

Studies on dogs have been done where the pericardium was removed and the dogs' hearts were defibrillated.[2] It was found that the pericardium dramatically increased how much energy was

Yin

Yin needed, whilst also reducing the number of hearts that recovered. There can be no doubt then that the pericardium is a very good electrical insulator or shield of the heart, but what this model proposes is something further…that the pericardium actively, consciously, shields the heart from electromagnetic forces.

Science fiction is a massive fan of such active shields, often known as 'force fields'. Rather than looking after our hearts they tend to protect spaceships from photon torpedoes or planetary bases from attack. Science reality has had a lot more trouble generating such fields, however, since electromagnetic energy is difficult to contain…for starters it travels at the speed of light. Scientists have obtained magnetic shielding, though, by using nano-crystalline grain structure ferromagnetic metal coatings to create *Faraday cages*. In our body, do we use nano-semicrystalline structure collagen fibres?

If the above seems tenuous then that is because it is. What we are talking about is how our bodies, mind and spirit interact with others, not on a physical level but on an emotional level. Emotions are beyond science; almost by definition people's emotional lives are irrational, so how can we expect science to provide a rational explanation for how they work?

Science isn't entirely rational, though. Chaos theory is the theory of tiny changes creating irrationally massive differences, and quantum theory uses irrational concepts to describe how tiny things behave (for instance, they flit in and out of existence!).

How and if the electromagnetic structure of the pericardium protects our heart and allows us to love our life and stay out of emotional mischief is a mystery, but it is getting awfully close to the meaning of life. Whilst the pericardium can be seen to shield the heart from electromagnetism – a coarse form of Qi – how does that work in a way that not only protects us but also provides our life with meaning? The science of this appears more metaphysics than physics, a problem for philosophers rather than physicists. It is beyond current science to explain why you fall in love with someone. Indeed, I hope it always is – some things are more beautiful as a mystery.

Despite the mystery, science can tell us something about at what level this is occurring. In the Chinese medical model, the vibrating semi-crystalline structure of the Pericardium enwraps the Heart. Electromagnetic energy from the Heart passes through this, and energy entering the Heart has to pass through the Pericardium to enter.

To all those nay-sayers out there who think this sounds ridiculous, it is no more ridiculous than finding there are parts of your house where your mobile phone has bad reception: the walls are preventing electromagnetic radiation from entering, meaning that you cannot communicate with your loved ones.

Imagine if the walls of your house were instead made of a very fine metallic mesh, like wire wool, with each fibre carefully laid down with an organic exactitude. Imagine further that the house was alive and every second it produced a powerful surge of electromagnetism, that this surge interacted with the house in ways that were poorly understood. Is it now so difficult to imagine that your cellular reception might depend on how your house was behaving, how it was *feeling*?

This interaction between waveforms occurs at an extremely subtle level, a level of science that is called the quantum level. This is the level at which our consciousness resides, as even many scientists accept that our brains are 'quantum computers'.[3] At this level, energy passing through structures affects their energy and interacts with them in strange ways. Amongst other things it can create resonance, and so when you get someone's vibe, or like their energy, you really are connecting at an energetic level. This is one reason why you can create such instantaneous impressions about people.

Post-script: One of the leading drugs for dealing with manic behaviour is lithium. Mania is seen as a problem with the Pericardium protecting the Heart in Chinese medicine. No one quite understands why lithium works, but for the above to be correct then lithium would also have to affect the electrical behaviour of collagen. Studies have shown that, at therapeutic levels, lithium does indeed affect collagen organisation and makes

Yin

Yin   the collagen fibrils smaller.[4, 5] I would theorise that further research would show that these changes also affect the electrical behaviour of collagen and account (at least in part) for lithium's effectiveness at controlling mania.

Arm JueYin – The Pericardium channel

The Pericardium channel is not much easier to understand than the organ.

When your body is a mere five weeks old (or roughly the size of the word 'embryo' on this page) it divides itself up internally, forming primitive chest and abdomen. The diaphragm is the part of the body that does this, and just to make things complicated it is composed of three separate embryological parts, all of which have horribly complicated names:

- the septum transversum

- the pleuropericardial folds, and

- the meso-oesophagus.

The names are not important, but what they do is:

- The septum transversum comes down from the throat area and forms the central part of the diaphragm that transmits the channels (otherwise known as the aorta, oesophagus and vena cava). It is also critical for making the liver grow and forms the ligaments between liver and stomach.

- The pleuro-pericardial folds grow out from the chest wall and form the thick fibrous pericardium. The fibrous pericardium forms from the tissue of the chest wall, and this is why the Pericardium Acupuncture channel starts on the chest wall.

- The meso-oesophagus surrounds the oesophagus.

These three fuse to form the diaphragm. The result is that the pericardium, liver, diaphragm and oesphageal sphincter are not only anatomically linked but also embryologically fused.

Yin

Again, it's easier to describe as the JueYin channel of Chinese medicine.

The JueYin is the Acupuncture channel that goes from the middle finger to the chest, enters the pericardium, crosses the diaphragm and then enters the liver. From here it passes down through the abdomen before emerging at the femoral canal to go down the inside of the leg.

The Chinese didn't really talk about the 'diaphragm' but they knew there was a 'greasy membrane' which divided the abdomen from the chest. The diaphragm is considered part of the Triple Burner, and the Pericardium is also part of this.

The similarity between the connections and organs formed by the embryological diaphragm and the channels and organs of the JueYin channel is not coincidence. They are the same thing!

What the ancients described in this Acupuncture channel complex makes no sense until you look at the embryology; then it appears as though it has been lifted from a textbook. The connections are all there in adult life, but they are not as obvious because they are purely fascial connections. Pericardium connects to the diaphragm through the phreno-pericardial ligaments that transmit the phrenic nerve amongst other things. Diaphragm and liver are connected through the bald patch of the liver.

The most famous function of the Pericardium channel is to treat nausea with the point found on the inside of the wrist – *Nei Guan* (Inner Gate) PC-6.

This point has been well studied. It is used by anaesthetists in the recovery room, sailors on rough voyages and many a pregnant woman with debilitating morning sickness. It is a favourite of Acupuncturists where its function is seen as more complex than subduing Rebellious Stomach Qi, the technical description for throwing up.

There is no compelling reason why this point should affect nausea, until you consider the embryology and fascia.

Yin

The reason that *Nei Guan* is called Inner Gate is that it enables connection to the corresponding Yang channel on the outside of the forearm.

These points are called *Luo* or Connecting points and allow pressure in the channels system to be transmitted from the Yin channels to the Yang (or vice versa).

The point lying across the forearm on the Triple Burner channel is known as *Wai Guan* TB-5, Outer Gate, and needling can open this gate allowing pathological Qi to move across. This is analogous to opening a flood gate to alleviate flooding.

We know this point works for nausea but up until now we could not explain why. What exactly is happening when you needle this point?

The pathways of Qi that connect *Nei Guan* PC-6 up through the fascia of the arm and into the armpit are easy enough to understand – they simply follow the fascial planes.

At the wrist these pass between the tendons of *flexor carpi radialis* and *palmaris longus*, continuing up to the elbow. At the elbow they continue onwards between the two heads of *biceps brachii*, following the short head to the *coracoid* process. Two muscles insert at the *coracoid* and the Qi follows the fascial plane around the second – the *pectoralis minor* muscle – down to the end of the muscle at the edge of the nipple.

The pericardium grows out of the chest wall early in embryogenesis and it is this connection that persists as the *sterno-pericardial ligaments*. Whilst these ligaments don't precisely match up with the nipple, they do provide a connection between pericardium and chest wall via the sternum. Furthermore, defects in pericardial development cause defects in the chest wall too,[1] so the connection between chest wall and pericardium is definitely there but the precise anatomy is elusive.

Needling *Nei Guan* PC-6 creates a fascial connection along this pathway that connects through the sterno-pericardial ligaments to the pericardium. The description is actually backwards since Qi is moving in the opposite direction, from areas of high to low pressure, from inside to out. Once this connection is made with the pericardium it is also connecting with the diaphragm and hence the liver, the central part of the diaphragm surrounding the oesphageal sphincter, and the fascial connection between liver and stomach.

In Chinese medicine, vomiting is often a product not of a Stomach problem but of an overactive Liver 'invading' the Stomach.

Needling *Nei Guan* PC-6 produces a precise fascial connection that moves along these planes of least resistance and connects them in the same way as fault lines link up on the Earth.

In the process of 'Liver Qi Invading Stomach and Rebelling Upwards' (another Chinese medicine description of throwing up), opening the channel through this pathway provides an outlet for this Qi so that it does not need to 'rebel'.

The name *Nei Guan*, Inner Gate, refers to its ability to open and release. This is a gate that is opened not to stop vomiting, for vomiting is caused by many different pathologies; it is a gate that releases the rebellious Qi in the JueYin.

This may not be correct, but it is the best explanation that you will currently find for why *Nei Guan* PC-6 helps vomiting.

Emergency case report

The Pericardium is a fantastic channel for nausea and I have often used it for this. It also helps gastritis and heartburn. I have also used it for a condition which is very difficult to treat well in Western medicine: pleurisy.

Pleurisy is an inflammation of the fascial lining of the lung. The pleura and pericardium are both fascial membranes in the chest, and when infection or irritation occurs in this space the pain is sharp and excruciating. A patient came into the department with exactly this pain.

Yin   The chest x-ray showed a tiny amount of infection in the lung corresponding to the area where she complained of the pain. The lung is insensitive to pain, so the pain came not from here but from the adjacent pleura becoming inflamed. The pain was severe and worse on breathing. Palpation of her channels showed lots of fine nodules at *Nei Guan* PC-6, and tenderness at *Chi Ze* (Cubital Marsh) Lu-5 and *Yin Ling Quan* (Yin Mound Spring) SP-9.

Massage at *Nei Guan* PC-6 and the corresponding Triple Burner point *Wai Guan* TB-5 caused her sharp pain to go completely. What was left was a dull ache (probably the sensation of fullness created by the infection in the lung). Massage of the Sea points of the TaiYin channel (*Yin Ling Quan* SP-9 and *Chi Ze* LU-5) helped the Qi to move in the right direction and almost completely cured this pain too. The patient was very happy and left with antibiotics to help clear the infection.

Even though the pericardium is distinct from the pleura, in this case it appeared that they were behaving as one. When the pericardium grows out of the chest wall it is continuous with the pleura at this point.[6] This connection will persist in some form and hence, from a Chinese medicine, Acupuncture and fascial point of view, the lung pleura is part of the Pericardium channel. This is why the Pericardium channel is useful in pleurisy.

The General

Yin

The Chinese saw the body as a reflection of our outer world – microcosm mirrored macrocosm. This concept produced many vivid illustrations of how our internal world reflected the world at large...

In our inner world, creation begins and the volcano of Ming Men erupts spewing lava (neural crest cells) into the primordial rivers of Yolk (TaiYin). Its explosive fire blasts out the pancreas, where at its apex a dusky blue mushroom cloud emerges – the Spleen.

Next to this, the Digestive Fire from Ming Men creates bubbling hot rivers of Yolk which overflow and course towards the outside. Here, where the Yolk and Fire mix and are cooled, the Liver forms, like a carpet of mangrove, and Blood is made.[*]

The alchemy of the body is almost complete – Yang forced its way into Yin causing the transformation of the Yolk Sac. To complete the circle of life, energy must return to Yang again.

The Chinese say that this occurs in the JueYin cavity in the body, where the Liver resides.

This word – JueYin – is comprised of two words: Jue and Yin.

Yin is self-explanatory. It is the feminine, dark, nourishing, yolky aspect of life.

Jue is formed from two aspects and has been a source of great confusion in Chinese medicine. The Tai in TaiYin is simple – it means greatest; likewise the Shao in ShaoYin simply means lesser. The Jue in JueYin is much more mysterious, though. Like all ancient Chinese it is helpful to look at the actual character:

---

[*] In the embryo the Liver not only makes many of the components of blood, but also makes the red blood cells too.

Yin   The first means a narrow opening in a mountainside, the second means an 'absence'. The JueYin is an opening in the mountainside where there is a passageway. This reflects the JueYin's role of returning Yin back to Yang.

(This description of a mountain pass is, as we shall see in 'The Lymph Channel' in Chapter 30, a very accurate description of the *actual* JueYin – a place in the body near the *cisterna chyli*.)

The *NeiJing SuWen* states that the Liver is the general, all orders emanate from it, and people who are felt to have a particularly strong Liver like to organise and make lists...

To-do list

Explain how:

- the Liver stores Blood
- Liver-Blood regulates menstruation
- the Liver ensures the smooth flow of Qi
- the Liver ensures the smooth flow of emotions
- the Liver hates Wind
- the Liver controls the Sinews.

The Liver stores Blood

In Chinese medicine the Liver stores Blood. The *SuWen* states that:[7]

> when a person lies down the blood returns to the liver.

Western medicine places much less emphasis on this property of the liver but still agrees with it wholeheartedly. At rest, the liver contains about 10–15 per cent of our blood, but when it is stimulated by bleeding or exercise it can contract and release about half a litre of blood into the circulation.[8, 9]

The liver is not only the largest organ in the body, it also *Yin* physically resembles a large clot of blood. Along with having its own blood supply from the heart, the entire blood of the digestive system drains into the liver and all the blood from below the diaphragm passes directly underneath it in the *vena cava*.

The extra blood the liver stores is extremely important during exercise and in Chinese medicine people who cramp up easily often have a deficiency of Blood.

East and West agree on this: the liver does store blood.

Liver-Blood regulates menstruation

When women have menstrual problems, Chinese medicine always looks to the Liver and specifically what it calls the *Liver-Blood*.

The liver is very important for the blood: it controls and makes the proteins, fats, cholesterol and clotting agents that are suspended in the blood. What these all share is that they are essentially insoluble in the watery part of the blood, they are fat-soluble and held in suspension. This is similar to how if you vigorously shake some water and oil mixed together it will make a creamy mixture – a suspension.

The liver controls the fatty aspect of our blood. For example, the kidney will eliminate most drugs but if it is fat-soluble it will have to be acted on by the liver first. Abnormal 'fatty' deposits in the body (atherosclerosis) caused by cholesterol are treated with statins – drugs that change how the liver processes this 'fat'.

When Chinese medicine talks about the Liver-Blood it is referencing this aspect of the Blood, the fat-soluble suspension that is under the control of the Liver. The rest of the blood consists of the water itself, ions and the red and white cells; as discussed, these are all under the control of the Kidney.

Clotting factors are the most obvious link between Liver-Blood and menstruation. Produced in the liver, these are critical for normal clotting and a disturbance in them can cause heavy bleeding. However, it is unusual to find any serious abnormality

Yin

when tests are done on women with heavy bleeding. Instead, when doctors treat abnormal menstrual bleeding the first line is invariably to use hormones to take control over the menstrual cycle. If this doesn't work with the 'Pill' then they will use progressively stronger hormones until eventually they induce an artificial menopause. Sledgehammers and nuts come to mind.

Another approach doctors use is a drug called *transexamic acid* which works by stopping clots being broken down. This works well but can cause blood clots elsewhere. Neither treatment really gets to the underlying pathology, though – instead, they are working around it.

In my work as a doctor I have met many women with painful and heavy periods, and I always recommend Acupuncture. Even simple massage at the point *San Yin Jiao* SP-6 is very effective. Part of the way in which it works is probably through the hormone *histamine*.

If there is one hormone that is associated with the liver, it is histamine. The liver is the primary organ for breaking histamine down:[10, 11] histamine is raised in liver disease;[12] and using antihistamines helps treat the symptoms of liver failure.[13] Histamine makes you irritable – allergies, rashes, hives and bites are all made itchy and irritable by histamine. In Chinese medicine the Liver also controls the *emotional aspects* of maintaining appropriate boundaries and anger; it is the organ of irritability. Histamine doesn't only make you feel irritable but also makes the body irritable against bugs and parasites. It marks out your own physical boundaries.

It should be no surprise then, to students of Chinese medicine, that women with dysfunctional uterine bleeding have raised levels of histamine in their wombs.[14] Histamine is contained within 'granules' in specialised cells called *mast cells*. At menstruation these mast cells 'degranulate' and release their histamine.[15] (Attentive readers may note that this is the same process as occurs in anaphylaxis.) At the risk of annoying 50 per cent or more of my readers, this is one reason why some women become…ahem…a little more irritable once a month.

Yin

Histamine doesn't just make women at their time of month irritable, it also causes the womb to be more leaky to red cells and fluid. Around 50 per cent of a woman's 'blood' loss is not blood at all: it is actually fluid that has leaked out,[15] and histamine makes this worse.

Histamine is one link between the liver and women's menstrual problems and it also links in with pre-menstrual syndrome (PMS). Many of the common symptoms of pre-menstrual syndrome – headache, insomnia, tiredness, nausea, abdominal pain, diarrhoea – are also linked to histamine intolerance.[16] Furthermore, asthma, urticaria,[17, 18] eczema[19] and epilepsy[20] have all been shown to get worse during PMS and these are conditions that have histamine and mast cells at their core (apart from epilepsy, which we will come to). Furthermore, many of the foods that women find make PMS worse – chocolate, red meat and alcohol – all contain either high levels of histamine or its culinary mother *histadine*.

It would be disingenuous to ignore the cyclical nature of menstruation, and we know that this cycle runs on oestrogen and progesterone. Many of the symptoms of PMS have (correctly or otherwise) been attributed to an imbalance of these two hormones, especially progesterone. Histamine and these hormones are linked, though: histamine increases progesterone levels,[21] and experts believe that mast cells become more active and numerous in the uterus in response to these two hormones.[22]

What this amalgam of East and West is proposing is that when the East states that the Liver regulates menstruation, one of the ways it does this is through the metabolism of the hormone histamine.

If mast cells and histamine lie near the root of women's monthly problems, curing them may not be as simple as using antihistamines. It has been known for over 70 years[23] that this same pathology often underlies asthma (in Chinese medicine this variant is seen as Liver Qi stagnation affecting Lungs), but antihistamines have had very little success here despite the fact that successful treatments reduce histamine levels.[24] Antihistamines are used in PMS – Midol™ being an example – but they are (currently) not a mainstay of treatment. A trial of antihistamines at the beginning of a woman's period would, however, be interesting…

Yin   The Liver ensures the smooth flow of Qi

There is little way to compare this to the Western view of the body because Western medicine ignores Qi.

Qi is organisational energy. When it is running in the Acupuncture channels it is extremely refined, but Qi is present everywhere in the body. It can be a bit confusing when translating to Western concepts as many different Western concepts are subsumed into Qi. Nerve energy too is a form of Qi, and emotions are a manifestation of Qi since emotions help organise our spirit.

Cramping abdominal pain is an example of Qi that is not moving smoothly, but so is feeling irritable and twitchy. Our spirit and mind reside in our body, and if our body is not at rest then neither can our minds be.

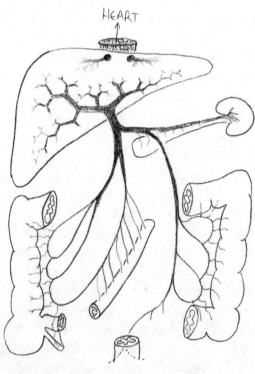

PORTAL CIRCULATION OF LIVER

The liver is not only an organ that stores blood but it is also a highly fascial organ. It is linked to every digestive organ in the abdomen through the *portal venous system*, and also the diaphragm, oesophagus, stomach and pancreas through ligaments. There are five ligaments that emerge from the liver, which is extraordinary for an organ.

The portal venous system is the blood, rich in absorbed nutrients from food, that goes from the gut to the liver without going through the heart first. Normally all the blood returns straight to the heart to be recycled, but in the digestive system it goes to the liver instead. The importance of this is that the liver gets to see everything you absorb from your food first.

Blood coming from the gut can contain many different things; any old junk that you have swallowed. It is vitally important that the liver gets to give this a clean first before it goes to your heart. Poisons can be detoxified, bacteria killed, fats made more mellow. This is part of the JueYin function of protecting the Heart.

When working well, the liver handles all this work with aplomb. However, if the liver is working slowly then this system gets backed up. In extremis, when the liver is failing the pressure in the portal system rises so much that the liver literally sweats out fluid into the peritoneum.

To non-medics,

'peritoneum'

probably means as much as

'monkey jo-jo numani'.

However, unlike 'monkey jo-jo numani', the peritoneum really exists.

The peritoneum is an enormous (potential) space in your abdomen. Practically all keyhole surgery on the abdomen is done in this space.

In liver disease, the peritoneum fills up with fluid – this is called *ascites*.

Ascites is an extreme example of Liver Qi and Blood stagnation. It only occurs when things have gone seriously wrong. The primary

Yin

Yin problem with ascites is often this build-up of pressure in the blood supply from gut to liver – *portal venous hypertension*. In Chinese terms the Liver is not helping the smooth flow of Blood and Qi from the digestive organs.

Smooth flow of Qi goes hand-in-hand with smooth flow of Blood, since Qi is the commander of Blood. In other words, organisational energy moves Blood around the body to where it is needed; where Qi goes, Blood follows.

If extremely stagnant Liver Qi and Blood cause a back-up of fluid in the peritoneum (ascites) then this tells us something important: the Liver keeps the fluid in the peritoneum flowing smoothly.

In fact, the Liver and the peritoneum are the same thing: the Liver controls the peritoneum. This makes the Chinese assertion that:

the Liver enables the smooth flow of Qi

make much more sense.

Qi flows in the fascial planes and the largest fascial plane in the body is the peritoneum. The Liver ensures that the peritoneum is clear of fluid by keeping the gut (portal) blood pressure low and so enabling the smooth flow of blood and Qi.

When working as a trainee surgeon (I gave it up when I realised I didn't have the dedication to be one), I once saw the bowels of a woman with IBS first-hand. The surgeon pointed out the oedema or swelling of the intestines and pressed on the gut, leaving a small indent where the fluid had been squeezed out.

'That,' he said, 'is common in IBS.' There was no follow-up to this: it was just a statement of fact.

One of the problems with Western medicine is its insensitivity, which often manifests in the language doctors use:

'There is nothing wrong' should actually be said as 'Our tests are too insensitive to find anything wrong.'

'There is no treatment for this' means 'There are no drugs or surgery I can give you which can fix the problem.'

IBS is an example. It is impractical to open up every IBS patient's abdomen to tell him or her that their guts are swollen, and it won't change anything, but none of our other tests will really do it. When patients with IBS complain that their belly feels bloated and swollen, they are not mad – their guts really are!

By the time that Liver Qi stagnation has become serious enough to cause ascites then it is pretty advanced, but there is a whole spectrum of Liver Qi stagnation that presents with just a little swelling and no ascites.

If *portal blood* flow is going slowly, sludgily, then it probably won't show up on any tests, but it will still be a problem. This sludgy flow will cause swelling of the tissues behind it and result in the gut becoming swollen.

This is what the Chinese were talking about when they said that:

the smooth flow of Liver Qi aids digestion

and why they often use the Liver when treating IBS.

Our old friend histamine pops up again. Histamine (or technically histidine) is produced in many foods, typically all the things that taste great – like matured cheese, wine and aged meats.

In fact, histamine is a marker of food going off and that is why you find it in all these aged foods. Histamine is also found in badly stored tuna fish, and when people eat this they can get a condition called 'scombroid poisoning' – throbbing headache, abdominal cramps, nausea and diarrhoea. All these symptoms Chinese medicine considers to be caused by Liver Qi stagnation with Heat, and what this displays is that sometimes the liver cannot deal with the amount of histamine that is absorbed and so it overflows into the blood.

The liver aids digestion in both East and West, but Chinese medicine is aware of a subtlety that is absent in Western medicine that emerges from the Liver not just taking all the blood from the gut, but also its Qi too…

Yin

Yin   ## The Liver ensures the smooth flow of emotions

The Liver Qi doesn't just enable smooth digestion – when it flows smoothly it also enables a smooth emotional state. We all know people who are tetchy and irritable. They rise easily to anger and are probably best left alone when they are having a bad day. The kind of people with anger that is always coming to the surface are seen as having a Liver problem in Chinese medicine.

Anger is difficult to pin down in terms of hormones. Oxytocin is thought to be the love hormone, serotonin the feel-good hormone, adrenaline the…well, adrenaline hormone, but anger has evaded easy classification. Partly this is because there are two main types – repressed anger and expressed anger – that depend on issues of social dominance and impulse control.

Ignoring the issue of dominance, anger often rises from frustration, and the sister of frustration is irritability. The next time you find yourself getting angry, stop and feel what is going on. Almost certainly there will be frustration and irritability, whether it is at a stuck drawer, a nagging partner or England's lack of ability to string more than a few passes together at football.

There is a hormone of irritability – it is histamine. Histamine is a hormone designed to make your body irritable against pathogens. It causes swelling, attracts white cells and generally is a good thing because it localises the pathogen and irritates your body against it. Histamine should really remain a localised hormone but sometimes the hormone can overflow in the system and cause the whole body to be irritable. Allergy, asthma, anaphylaxis all have histamine overload. The hallmark of histamine is itch, and an itch you can't scratch is almost the definition of irritability and frustration.

The Liver's ability to ensure the smooth flow of emotions relies upon its ability to clean the blood of histamine and other related substances. It might not always be histamine; it just so happens that whenever the functions of the Chinese Liver are discussed, Western medicine places a central role with histamine but there are certainly other chemicals involved in irritability. In some ways it possibly should be the concept of Histamine rather than histamine.

Yin

The Liver hates Wind

Wind is a pathogenic factor in Chinese medicine, a concept of something ephemeral that gets into the body and injures it.

In nature, wind moves and changes direction quickly. In the body, like Qi, pathogenic Wind is insubstantial. As in nature it arises from heat, creates movement and can be destructive.

Wind is an enemy of Qi, because it can move Qi around easily – Qi is ethereal and insubstantial too and so Wind easily affects it. The Chinese used the metaphor of Wind to describe the type of illnesses that afflicted the body in a similar way: epilepsy, tics, tremors, shaking, urticaria and afflictions that move around the body are all 'Wind'.

If you look at the Western interpretations of these types of illnesses they are mainly *neurological* in nature – in other words, problems of electrical energy in the nerves. Only with extremely sensitive tests that detect changes in electricity can Western medicine find any pathology. Epilepsy can be measured with the energy detected by an EEG; most tremors are considered to be 'essential' – a short form of 'essential-ly no idea why they are happening'; 'tics' often elude capture; and urticaria is a disease that is treated rather than understood.

What these conditions all share is that there is little substantial change to the body. In a heart attack you can physically see the damaged heart; likewise in bronchitis, or stomach ulcers or even kidney inflammation (if you go to the trouble of taking a sample of kidney). In epilepsy an EEG doesn't see the pathologic injury; it just sees the aberrant energy (Wind) moving around. When Chinese medicine talks about Wind, Western science agrees: it is a condition of abnormal movement of energy.

All these conditions are seen as a manifestation of Wind, and the Chinese consider Wind to be most serious when it enters the

Yin   Blood level of the body – the deepest energetic level of the body. The Liver is seen as being rich in Blood, responsible for storing the Blood, and ultimately for eliminating this Wind. Epilepsy is one of the most dramatic and obvious examples of Wind, Wind that has entered the Blood level of the body.

It is very interesting, then, that one of the most common side-effects (the medical establishment often uses this word as a synonym for poisoning, but in this case it truly is a side-effect) of anti-epileptics is that they induce liver enzymes. This side-effect is considered particularly troubling because it causes the liver to detoxify other drugs and sometimes even the anti-epileptic drug faster than normal. Vast amounts of money have been spent trying to find anti-epileptics that do not have this effect, with some limited success, but a student of Chinese medicine will tell you that it is precisely because of this effect that they are so effective as anti-epileptics: the drugs are inducing the Liver to metabolise Wind faster.

We sometimes know what triggers epilepsy: there can be abnormal spots in the brain that create aberrant energy. What we don't really understand is why that goes on to cause epilepsy.

Neurons are supposed to be inherently stable. They have mechanisms for preventing random mischief-makers from dragging the rest into epilepsy, but in some people's brains this doesn't happen. Many people have damage to their brain and never get epilepsy; others apparently have no damage but get it all the time. What is now being implicated is damage to the blood–brain barrier (BBB) – the membrane that acts to prevent noxious substances from getting into the brain.[25] The barrier is there to protect the brain: only carefully controlled substances can pass across it.

The relationship between blood and brain is incredibly intimate, yet also deliberately distant. There are thought to be 100 billion capillaries in the brain, one for every neuron, but the actual blood is kept separate from the neurons. The capillaries' cells are tightly woven together to prevent anything leaking through. What a lot of research is suggesting is that we are moving from a model

Yin

where epilepsy is a condition of the brain to a model where it is a condition of the blood or substances within it leaking into the brain.

The 'brain' is really two organs in one. There is the enormous network of blood that supplies it but is distinct from it, and the neurons that produce all the electricity. This is an example of Blood nourishing Qi. So, when the Chinese say that Wind in the Blood causes conditions like epilepsy, they may just be right; it is just a question of interpretation.

One hormone that is absolutely known to damage the BBB is – surprise, surprise – histamine. In fact: 'Histamine is one of the few central nervous system neurotransmitters found to cause consistent blood–brain barrier opening.'[26] Histamine is the hormone of irritation: it keeps you awake at night, makes your skin itchy, your breathing wheezy, your eyes red, gives you heartburn and generally makes you tetchy. Histamine makes your neurons alert, but, in health, histamine doesn't cross from blood to neurons but instead works on the BBB.

Strangely, histamine has two opposite effects on the barrier depending on which receptor it activates. If it activates H1 (the same receptor that is knocked out by hay fever medications) then the barrier is less permeable; if it activates H2 (the receptor that is knocked out by heartburn medications) it is more permeable.[26] Drugs that knock out the H1 receptor do indeed make epilepsy worse and trigger fits in febrile children, whereas drugs that knock out H2 don't, and also make the liver work faster (and in fact, I would hypothesise, will be anti-convulsant).

The links between the liver and seizures (Wind) don't end there.

In liver failure people become brain-sick (encephalopathic), and as the liver fails toxins build up that cause the person to become irritable and twitchy. The first sign of this brain-sickness is sleep disturbance, and antihistamines are effective at treating this.[7] As the liver disease gets worse these toxic compounds build up in the blood and the irritability becomes worse. Histamine is not the only chemical that will cause brain irritability, but it acts as a marker of liver dysfunction.

Yin   In rats that were made encephalopathic (possibly by being forced to watch re-runs of England's 2010 World Cup matches), histamine was found to be significantly raised in their brains.[27]

Eventually, liver failure causes seizures in up to 50 per cent of patients.[28] This predilection towards seizures is not seen to the same extent with failure of other organs.

The Liver controls the Sinews

Thankfully this has nothing to do with histamine…as far as we know. Sinews are the parts of the body that enable flexibility; they are the tendons and ligaments and even the connective tissue within muscles that keep them from breaking.

Weak sinews presents with snapped tendons, tight tendons or ripped muscles. What is being shown is that these are weak and prone to rupture because of abnormal cholesterol metabolism.[29]

The Liver of Western medicine and Chinese medicine are thus not that different; they actually agree on all the main points. Whilst Western medicine sees the liver primarily as an organ of poison detoxification, protein and clotting formation and assisting in digestion, Chinese medicine sees it as an organ of detoxification of Wind, smooth flow of Blood and Qi, and assisting in digestion. The difference is in the details and how this is seen to function.

Furthermore, the absence of Qi within Western medicine does not allow for connections in Acupuncture theory that become self-evident when considering the fascia and embryology.

Leg JueYin – The Liver channel

In English football there has only ever been one general. I raise my glass to the inestimable gentleman of sport, a prince of the public, and a general of football – Sir Bobby Charlton.

Yin

Bobby Charlton, as a great midfielder, was able to distribute the ball where it was needed, when it was needed. From the middle of the pitch he had connections to all the players – defence, attack and the rest of midfield. In this way he was able to direct play and act like a general.

The Liver also has this role: it has connections to all the organs through the peritoneum and so can direct play (Qi) as needed. Strangely, Bobby Charlton doesn't just resemble the functions of the Liver, but also the anatomy.

You see, just like Bobby Charlton, on the uppermost part of the liver is the anatomical *bald area.** Unlike Bobby Charlton's bald area, there is no comb-over but instead there sits a crown.

The 'crown' is called the coronary ligament (I was surprised to find coronary is Latin for 'crown', not 'heart' as I had always presumed) and is formed by the peritoneum.

Imagine you are watching Bobby Charlton's majestic head slowly rise out of a calm lake. Before you can see his eyes, you see where a crown would sit…that is what the bald area looks like.

Now, presuming Bobby can still hold his breath, the water around his head represents the *peritoneal reflections*, and the whole of it forms a circle. This circle is the *coronary ligament*. Now transfer this to the underside of the diaphragm; this is the connection between liver and pericardium (via diaphragm).

Now take Bobby out, give him a warm towel and a pint of ale… My God, man! What were you thinking of, the man is a legend!

Surgeons think the bald area is important because it represents a point where infection can move from abdomen to thorax; the body thinks it's important because it enables communication between diaphragm and liver.

This communication is surprisingly vital, for the liver has to be directed in its development by part of the diaphragm – the *septum transversum*.

---

*　Strictly speaking this is called the *bare* area.

Yin   Even though the liver grows out of the Yolk Sac of the embryo, it needs the primitive diaphragm to direct it. This connection will persist in adult life and the bald area is a reflection of this.

When I was 32 I went to see an Acupuncturist for heart palpitations. She cured them and then set to work on other stuff. One treatment she gave left me actually feeling my diaphragm for the first time. I physically felt it loosen, which I was quite astonished by because I had never even been aware it was there before. I was able to breathe deeply again and felt relaxed and high.

When I remarked on this she replied with a knowing smile, 'That is the JueYin. It connects to the diaphragm through Liver and Pericardium.'

As a doctor I thought: 'Err, what are you talking about?'

Now it seems obvious: it's all in our embryology. The pericardium and diaphragm are formed from the same embryological beginnings that control liver growth and create its connective tissue – growth induced by the septum transversum, fusing with the pleuropericardial folds. These are the same folds that then make the pericardium.

Describing it as the JueYin channel just makes it easier to say!

This is the direction the Liver channel takes upwards, to connect with Pericardium through the diaphragm, but which direction does it go downwards?

It doesn't. Just as Acupuncture theory boringly teaches, it goes in all directions. This is why it is called *the general* because it organises so much. Liver Qi actually takes a multitude of directions through its multiple fascial connections.

If these fascial connections could be summed up in one word, though, it would be 'monkey jo-jo numani'. Sorry…'peritoneum'.

The peritoneum connects with almost everything in the abdomen, and the liver is responsible for keeping this fluid clear and enabling circulation which ends at the real JueYin (see Chapter 30 to find out where this is).

The bottom part of the peritoneum laps over the rectum, the ovaries, fallopian tubes and womb, and then the bladder.

Then it does something unusual in women – it connects to the
outside world via the fallopian tubes.

Yin

The fallopian tubes are named after an(other) Italian anatomist
called Gabriele Falloppio, but they have a more musical name from
the Greek for trumpet – *salpinx*. They were named after a trumpet
because they look like one, and the fat loud end opens into the
peritoneum and catches any eggs released by the ovaries.

This connection between liver, peritoneum and trumpets is
intriguing because Chinese medicine places great importance on
the Liver and women's parts. The Liver Qi is felt to circulate around
the pelvic organs in much the same way in which the peritoneum
folds over these organs. In the case of excessive vaginal discharge it
is almost always considered to be a problem involving pathological
Liver Yin! The Chinese would consider that the peritoneal fluid
(Liver Yin) is almost physically leaking down into the trumpets.

Western medicine makes this connection too, but in a
backwards way. There is a condition called *Fitz-Hugh–Curtis
syndrome* which somewhat bizarrely is classically (i.e. 10–15% of
the time) associated with water-skiing accidents!

On these occasions high pressure water can be forced up into
a woman's bits…ouch…and if that area is colonised by certain
unsavoury characters…'Chlamydia Pissartist' and 'John O'Rhea'…
then these can be forced backwards into the peritoneum.

From here the bugs move up to the liver where they set
up home creating the characteristic signs of *Fitz-Hugh–Curtis
syndrome* – liver adhesions (or Phlegm). The water-skiing example
is a rather graphic description, but the same process can happen
for no clear reason and illustrates the intimate link between these
two, apparently distinct, organs – the liver and uterus.

Liver and peritoneum are undoubtedly linked, but fascial
Qi theory teaches that Qi cannot cross fascia – it is the bedrock
around which organisation is formed. The peritoneum is a closed
sac of fascia… How can Liver Qi get in?

The liver (and odd organ) is *fenestrated* – this is practically
the only place in the body where blood mingles with the cells
without any barrier. The energy from Ming Men has been mixed

Yin   with Blood, it has been forced up through muddy waters and now is combining to form great blooms of green.

These blooms of green form a subtle liquid, like the evaporation from trees. The fluid oozes from every part of the peritoneum, but it starts at the liver and works its way round to the actual JueYin (see Chapter 30).

The Liver Qi controls the circulation in the peritoneum, and the peritoneum has only two other exits out of the abdomen.

These exits are weak spots where the bowel can sometimes push through and are the inguinal and femoral canal.

The inguinal canal is the part of the Liver channel that the ancient Chinese medical classics describe as going down to circulate around the testes and scrotum. This spot is a natural plane of least resistance (remember that Qi flows down pathways of least resistance) and is the most common place for hernias.

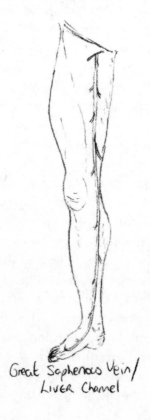

Great Saphenous Vein/
LIVER Channel

Likewise, the femoral canal is the exact spot where the ancient Chinese classics describe the Liver channel emerging into the leg. Deadman[30] describes it thus:

> *Jimai* (Rapid Pulse) Liv-12 is then located just medial to the vein on the groin crease.

This is equally the description of the femoral canal.

These are continuations of the peritoneum into the testes and leg respectively.

At the leg the rest of the channel is easy – it follows the lymphatics around the great saphenous vein, as shown in the figure.

Emergency case report

The Liver channel is often used for painful conditions since it enables the smooth flow of Qi.

Pain is considered to be a blockage of Qi, possibly caused by other things such as trauma, stagnant Blood or Phlegm, but ultimately all leading to a blockage of Qi.

A woman came into the department with trigeminal neuralgia. Trigeminal neuralgia is a horrible disease that consists of sharp pains like needles in the face. It is named after the trigeminal nerve that it affects. She had tried the normal painkillers, but this disease is immune to painkillers and requires toxic and dangerous drugs like carbamazepine and gabapentin. I counselled her for this, explained that we would need to check her blood since these drugs can cause anaemia and liver problems. Then I realised – at that point, in that hospital – that my seniors allowed me to use Acupuncture and asked her if she would like to try it.

Of course she agreed!

The nurses were curious and I was nervous. What happened if it didn't work – I would look very foolish with my quackery. The points I used were local points in the face and then some on the arm to help move the Qi, but I also used the point *Tai Chong*

Yin

Yin   (Great Rushing) Liv-3 in combination with *He Gu* (Joining Valley) LI-4.

The combination of these points is called the four gates and this opens the channels of Qi to allow it to flow.

In retrospect I didn't fully understand what I was doing with these points but the results were spectacular. Of course, there was nothing to see…apart from an elated patient. She practically danced out of the department after being free of pain for the first time in a week.

Some of the nurses were very impressed, but clearly others thought that I'd overstepped some boundaries…

Sadly, this case and others gave the medical establishment in the Emergency Department the willies. Not because anything bad happened – quite the reverse – but because something could have, and it would leave me open to criticism. My consultants pointed out there would be very few people to defend me and I had to accept their point – they had my best interests at heart and I stopped using the needles, but continued to use acupressure.

Instead of needles I went back to the 'safe' practice of draining blood, placing needles the size of knitting needles in chests, and giving medicines that could cause brain haemorrhages, stomach ulcers or heart attacks on the statistical probability that it would do good. Those medicines had powerful drug companies behind them that would defend them, and hence me.

Medicine is ruled by drug companies whose primary motivation is profit. They distort the entire system, they fund the research, they (indirectly) choose the professors – in effect they rig the system. Until people realise what a distorted, corrupted place the health system and medical 'research' is, then we are not going to get the best out of it.

The Three Yang Channels

The three internal pathways that wrap the six Yin organs are thus formed.

The Yang channels are much simpler. This is because the Yang organs are hollow. Hollow organs are also *channels* and so the Yang organ and channel are the same thing.

Again, these three channels each have a Yin and a Yang end, and an arm and a leg end:

- Bladder and Small Intestine form *TaiYang*

- Stomach and Large Intestine form *YangMing*

- Gallbladder and Triple Burner create *ShaoYang*.

28

TaiYang (Greater Yang)

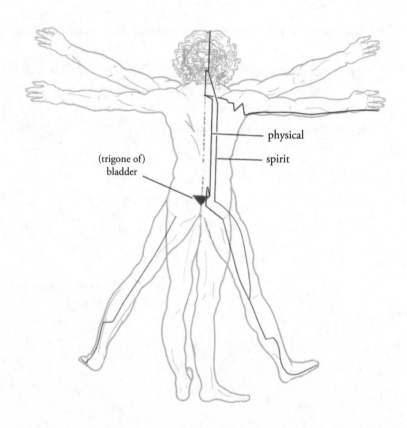

physical

spirit

(trigone of)
bladder

The Surfing Channel   *Yang*

The Bladder channel starts at the eye, runs behind the head and then divides to run down the back in four lines before it goes down the leg. It is easily the longest channel in the body (see the illustration on the previous page).

These lines correspond to the fascial planes between the muscles that run up behind the spine.

What is different about the Bladder channel is that all the points running alongside the spine are not named in relation to their effect on the bladder, but on their adjacent organ: this starts with the Lung at *Fei Shu* (Lung Shu) BL-13, and then runs through each and every organ to end (appropriately enough as we shall see) with the Bladder organ at *Pang Guang* (Bladder Shu) BL-28.

All these points are even named after their respective organ Lung Shu, Spleen Shu…and the eminent Dr Wang Ju-Yi believes these points are best for treating physical problems in the organ. Lateral to this lies the other line of Bladder points and these are named after the *spirit* of their respective organ; these are good for the spiritual (psycho-emotional) aspect of the organ.

To understand where this mysterious and enigmatic channel came from, we have to go back to the beginning of the Kidney, before even Ming Men, to the age of the Middle-kidneys (about 25 days).

The Middle-kidneys emerge at the same time as the heart, when our body is just a tiny embryo, along the back of our body as a paired line of:

> …swellings from the upper thoracic region to the lumbar spine.[1]

Yang

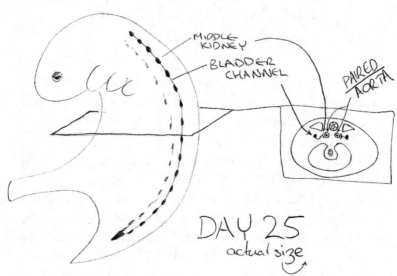

Each Middle-kidney connects to a 'tube' which runs alongside the developing spine to drain into the Yolk Sac via what will become the back of the bladder (little triangle at the end of the two lines near the tail in the picture). This 'tube' is a bladder! The Middle-kidneys are functioning and vital, as they are the only kidneys we have until ten weeks.

The Bladder channel of Chinese medicine thus corresponds almost perfectly with the 'bladder' of these primitive Middle-kidneys.

These Middle-kidneys are tiny and lie in a line along the back in a space between what will become the muscles of the back (*paraxial mesoderm*) and the part of the embryo that will go on to form our inner organ cavities (the *lateral plates*). They function as perfect little kidneys, which means they have a collecting duct, nephron and therefore a connection to the aorta.

And what moves from the skin on our back to this space between aorta, Middle-kidneys and spine?

The coolest cells in embryology: the *neural crest cells*, of course!

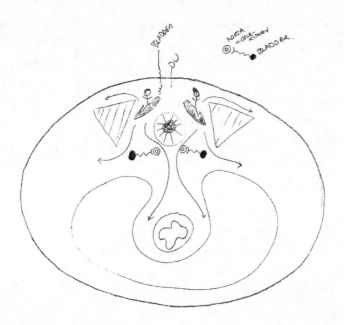

This is where they divide themselves up. When they surf out of that awesome barrel that is going to form your spinal canal, they're feeling good and they're going to get lucky. These cells will go and direct everything important in the body – they will *organise the organs*.

Some peel off to the side first and these correspond to the spirit points. The ones that delve straight into the interior are the physical back-shu points.

And this is why Dr Wang Ju-Yi states that these points are good for the physical organ: it is a reconnection between the neural crest cells and the organ they formed.

The relevance of this should be apparent. Here we have an exact anatomical and embryological correlate with the Bladder channel of Chinese medicine. Not only does it provide evidence of a physical connection in a line along the back to the bladder, but in a double line if you look at how this space connects with the back.

Unlike, for instance, the Lung channel, this channel cannot be seen in the adult because it disappears after around seven weeks, but it will still exist. If we carefully dissected the tissues of our back at a cellular level, we would find this primitive bladder in

Yang the same way that archaeologists find long-lost civilisations buried under jungles.

What this means is that placing a needle into this space reawakens these connections: it re-enforces the connection between neural crest cells, 'bladder' and organ. It is Acupuncture that is more like stem cell therapy, because really that is what Acupuncture is: the cheapest stem cell therapy you'll ever get.

The Invisible Channel

The Small Intestine channel is interestingly named, because there are no clinical uses for it that involve the small intestine. The channel is almost exclusively used for problems in the channel fascia itself and is probably the pre-eminent channel to be used in neck problems. It is another channel that appears to have been misnamed.

Its connections to the neck occur via the upper end of the Bladder channel in a similar manner – remember it is the same channel, but just the upper aspect. It probably affects the emptying of the small intestine via the Heart through the invisible ligament – the Ligament of Treitz. This ligament actually has muscle fibres in it and can speed up and slow down the degree of emptying of the *12 inches of power* into the small intestine.

I knew a doctor who actually managed to force his small intestine up around his heart in a kiteboarding accident. Despite being obscenely intelligent he walked around like this for a few days complaining of chest pain before collapsing and almost dying! He told me that not a lot of doctors even know the two are connected – I think this must be the connection he is talking about.

Here's another picture of Ming Men (labelled in the illustration as ampulla of vater):

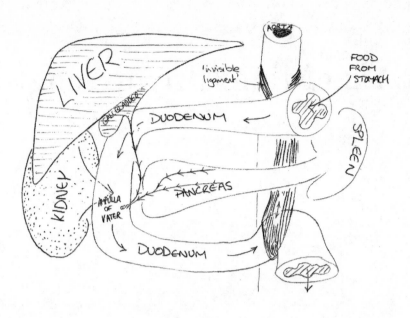

Emergency case report

In practice, I use the Yang channels a lot more than the Yin channels. This is because these channels are good for releasing excess and hence more apt for use in the Emergency Department.

The Bladder and Small Intestine channels are the pre-eminent channels to be used in back pain – I use them all the time in the Emergency Department. I particularly like the combination for acute back pain, as prescribed by Dr Wang Ju-Yi: *Jin Men* (Golden Gate) BL-63 and *Yang Gu* (Yang Valley) SI-5.

The Small Intestine channel is also very useful for neck problems and massage around the wrist area (SI-3–5), whilst getting the patient to move their neck resolves stiffness.

29

YangMing (Bright Yang)

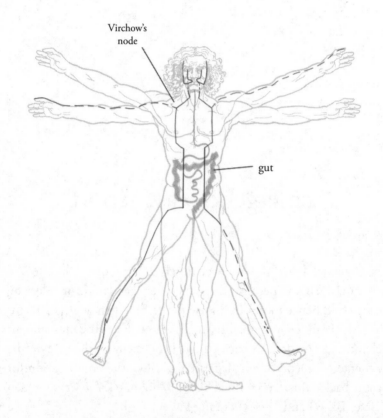

Virchow's node

gut

The Gut Channel

The Stomach in Chinese medicine is a much more vital piece of kit than the Western stomach. It is where the food is rotted and ripened, where the five grains are tasted, and the origin of all the fluid in our body.

There is a little problem reconciling this with the West, as these are not descriptions of what we describe as the stomach. Rather, this is a description of the entire alimentary system – what is commonly known as the gut.

The gut is simply a long tube. It begins at your mouth and ends at your rectum and in between lies a composting machine. The composting begins in the mouth where teeth break the food into smaller pieces allowing more contact with the composting juices. The mix is then swallowed, bypassing the lung at the voice box, and then smoothly passes down into the stomach.

The stomach works as the holding pen, slowly releasing the gloopy blend of food into the small intestine when it is ready. Like anywhere where you store food, bugs can be a problem, so acid is pumped in to kill them. The stomach contains a slimy surface that in health prevents acid eroding the stomach lining.

The small intestine is where the business end of composting lies. After entering the duodenum the food is mixed with enzymes secreted from the pancreas. These enzymes are incredibly powerful at breaking down proteins, starch, coffee, strawberry juice and chocolate, which is why scientists copied them and added them to washing powder.

At this point the gallbladder is also brought into play. Fats entering the small intestine trigger hormones, which cause the gallbladder to contract and release bile. The bile serves a number of purposes but the main one is to emulsify fats. Emulsification causes fats to be soluble in water, a process that enables the fat to be broken down into small enough particles to be absorbed. Again, scientists stole the same process and used it to make washing liquids that love greasy dishes.

Yang   The end result of this is that by the time your food has navigated the 30-odd feet of curled-up small intestine, it has become a broth. Most of the goodness has been absorbed: minerals, vitamins, sugars, proteins, fats. What remains is mainly water but a very large proportion of the rest is bacteria.

The bacteria will be immensely important in the last section of bowel – the large bowel. Vitamin means vital-amine/protein. By definition the body cannot make its own vitamins, but two of the vitamins are made inside the body, in the gut, by bacteria.

The reason vitamin K is called vitamin K is because the initial discoveries were reported in a German journal, in which it was named Koagulations vitamin. The Swedish scientist Pauling, who discovered vitamin K, knew it was essential for clotting – vitamin K is involved in making the clotting factors in the liver. One drug used to thin blood in patients is called warfarin and it is also rat poison; it stops these vitamin-K-dependent clotting factors being produced, but because this takes a few days the rats scamper off and die elsewhere. Rats die a horrible bloody death, but humans are monitored closely to prevent this.

Certain bacteria in the gut make vitamin K, and when people are on warfarin and take antibiotics they have to be careful. Antibiotics will kill the beneficial bacteria leading to less vitamin K and as a result the warfarin will work more strongly and become more (rat) poison, less medicine.

The other vitamin that is made is called biotin, and this too relies upon bacteria in the gut.

Bacteria get a bad press but the truth is that without them we are screwed. By the time the composting is done, one-third of the dry weight of your faeces is bacteria! We rely on them to not only create vitamins but also help break down the food and control growth of harmful organisms. Encouraging bacteria is one of the prime roles of the gut and it is not surprising that antibiotics wreak such havoc on gut health.

Apart from making hormones, the main role of the large intestine is in regulating the amount of fluid released at the other end. It is in the large intestine that the watery slop that emerges from our small intestine is slow cooked, dried and composted into *Yang* warm, moist pellets of manure, known to you and me as 'shit'.

The gut then is really one organ – a composting machine. Food goes in, gets broken down into a watery slop, has its goodness taken out, gets dried and then excreted the other end as compost/manure/shit. This process is extremely important and primal to our existence – without it we would die a slow lingering death. Chinese medicine holds that after birth it is this system that is the key to our health; however, it is not so much that you are what you eat as you are what you take from what you eat.

We know what happens when your stomach is removed. If you survive the operation and the reason for having it removed, then you can live a normal-ish life with smaller portion sizes. It is probably worse to lose your large intestine and have chronic diarrhoea, or your small intestine and suffer bodily wasting, than to lose your stomach.

When the Chinese described the Stomach as the origin of fluids they cannot mean the stomach of Western medicine – either that or they are mistaken. The stomach of Western medicine is a holding pen, it absorbs almost nothing; in fact, it probably secretes more fluid into the food in the form of acid than it takes back. Furthermore, the lining of the stomach is thick and viscous, designed to prevent its acidic contents from eroding it and in the process preventing absorption.

By contrast, the lining of the small intestine is a million miles of fronds, fractally built upon themselves. At each level of the fractal there is more surface area, so that the absorptive capacity of the small intestine is immense. This enormous amount of contact allows good things to be absorbed at the molecular level. Likewise, the large intestine is where most of the absorption of fluid occurs, not the stomach.

The 'Stomach' is therefore a misnomer. If the stomach was the origin of fluids, then removing it would be devastating – patients would have to be on lifelong intravenous fluids. This doesn't happen because it is the entire gut that is the origin of fluids, not the stomach.

Yang

When Chinese medicine talks of the Stomach, we have a problem of interpretation. The 'Stomach' is not the 'stomach' at all, it is the gut.

When put like that, the Chinese description of the 'Stomach' makes far more sense:

- The gut is the origin of fluids.

- The gut controls the rotting and ripening of the food.

Semantics are important. If sheep farmers and cow farmers cannot agree on whether a sheep is a called a sheep or a cow then butchers on Brick Lane will end up calling a cow a lamb (the butchers in Brick Lane know what I'm talking about). The same applies to medicine: if traditional Chinese Acupuncture practitioners are calling the 'gut' the 'Stomach' then it is no surprise that there is incredulity about its functions. The Stomach as origin of fluids?!

I couldn't find a name to describe the 'odd organ' earlier, but this one is easy: it should be called *the Gut*.

When the Stomach is talked about as the Gut, the nature of the Stomach becomes much clearer. It becomes so much clearer that from now on I will describe it as the Gut.

Yang within Yin

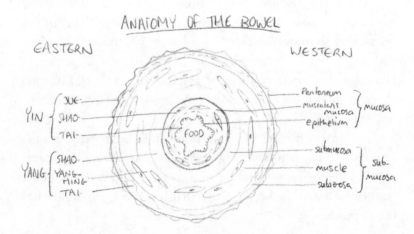

Anatomists have conveniently divided up the gut into six layers, which dovetails nicely with our six channels.

Furthermore they went to the trouble of subdividing these into two groups: mucosa and submucosa. Strangely, this fits perfectly with the Yin and Yang layers of Chinese medicine. (Well, perhaps it isn't really strange when you consider they are describing the same thing.) These layers are, from outside to inside:

- *Mucosa:*
  - Peritoneum (JueYin).

Then move to Yang:

- *Submucosa:*
  - Thick tough connective tissue, like skin (TaiYang).
  - Thick muscle which is rich in Qi and Blood (YangMing).
  - Lymphatic drainage (ShaoYang).

And then back to Yin:

- *Mucosa:*
  - Very sensitive muscle like the heart (ShaoYin).
  - Glands (Yolk Sac/TaiYin).

The Gut is a microcosm of our external layers but it lies internally. This is why instead of having skin (TaiYang) on its surface, it has glands – serosa (JueYin).

The Gut is *Yang within Yin.*

The whole Gut behaves like one fascial plane that starts at your mouth and ends at your arse. In between it weaves between TaiYin (anterior pararenal) and JueYin (intraperitoneal) as it moves down the body:

- the oesophagus is in TaiYin
- the stomach is in JueYin
- the duodenum is in TaiYin
- the small intestine is in JueYin

Yang

Yang

- the ascending colon is in TaiYin

- the transverse colon is in JueYin

- the descending colon is in TaiYin

- the sigmoid colon is in JueYin, and then finally

- the rectum is in the ShaoYin (it's in the pelvis).

This weaving of the actual Gut between JueYin and TaiYin accounts (in part) for why the Gut *channel* (uniquely) weaves across the TaiYin and JueYin channels.

The Yolk Sac forms the innermost of the cells, while the Gut is there to surround and protect it.

The Gut is best seen as a long muscular tube that has been invaded to varying degrees by the Yolk Sac. In parts this invasion is dramatic and forms entire organs such as the liver and pancreas; in other parts it is subtle and forms microscopic structures such as the *goblet cells* of the stomach (which secrete mucus to protect it from acid).

The muscular portion serves to move and protect; the glandular portion serves to lubricate and digest.

The part of the body that Chinese medicine recognises as the Gut is the muscular, Yang portion of the gut. This part of the body encircles the Yolk Sac in much the same way as the skin encircles the entire body.

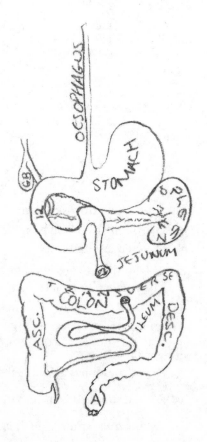

When this occurs it drags with it a blood and nervous supply *Yang* and these persist throughout life. This attachment is called the mesentery and it anchors all of the JueYin part to the back of the body.

Facial tectonics

Any surgeon will tell you that the mesentery is very important, not only as a rich seam of questions for unprepared medical students, but also for getting access to internal organs. The small intestine, attached as it is with a long mesentery, can be pulled out of the belly leaving a mass of entrails. Whenever you see a lion pawing through the guts of a zebra, or a dead whale's guts spilling onto a beach, it is the mesentery that enables this freedom of movement. (Incidentally, lions and other big cats always eat the glandular organs such as liver and pancreas of a kill before the muscles since they are much richer and more nutritious.)

The mesentery allows movement and provides attachment to the back.

The mesentery attaches at the midline, which is why even though the gut occupies almost the entirety of the abdomen, its connection to the rest of the body is very simple and lies down the middle at the front of our back.

The Gut channel, however, lies on the front, either side of the midline. It starts at the corners of our mouth and immediately branches to send a small branch to our eyes.

What is unusual about the Gut channel is that it is a Yang channel, but it is at the front of the body. In order to understand how this channel can be related to the gut we have to understand the embryological folding.

What we see as the face is actually an incredibly complicated formation. The reason that so many people who have developmental problems often have funny-looking faces (*dysmorphic* features) is that the face acts as a barometer of the developmental intelligence of the organism.

Yang   The face is a landscape of mountains (nose) and fiery lakes (eyes), forests (hairline) and cliff faces (cheekbones), and it does all this whilst maintaining balance and harmony.

No other part of the body contains so much variability, so many contrasts – and to create this reflects enormous organisational intelligence. The reason we look to the face for beauty (and romantic love) is because the beauty reflects health, and a health that is more than skin deep. High cheekbones and strong jawbones are not just prerequisites for being on the cover of *Vogue*, they also reflect the embryological equivalent of perfectly executed handbrake turns and double somersaults with pike.

The folding involved in the face is complicated but it revolves around three primary spots:

- the eye

- the mouth and nose

- the ear.

These three spots act as anchor points: they remain immobile while everything moves around them. They are immutable. They are also areas where the inside (Yolk Sac) meets the outside (Angmion) and it is therefore no surprise that all the Acupuncture channels on the face gravitate towards them and then end there:

- *The eye:* The Gut and Gallbladder (twice) channels go here and the Bladder channel ends here.

- *The mouth and nose:* The Gut channel starts here, and the Large Intestine channel ends at the nose.

- *The ear:* The Small Intestine, Triple Burner and Gallbladder channels all start/end here.

The channels all gravitate towards these spots precisely because they are singularities in the organism: they are points where the external and the internal meet; they are immutable, the folding occurs around them and they are spots where the internal and external Qi meet.

Yang

The Stomach channel has two branches on the face and one main channel. The main channel goes from the mouth, along the jaw and down the neck in what is an external reflection of the internal passage of the mouth into the throat and down the oesophagus.

The first branch goes from mouth to eye and the second branches up from the end of the jaw to pass up the side of the face ending at the 'corner of the head'. These branches reflect the fissures in the face as it forms. These fissures are formed between what are called the facial plates. The facial plates fit together rather in the same way as tectonic plates fit together to form the Earth. The fault lines between these tectonic plates in the face are the Acupuncture channels.

The facial plates start life as rather uninteresting blobs but will eventually form all our features. One example of failure of the facial plates to fuse properly is a cleft lip, where a gap remains between nose and mouth.

Que Pen's node

In the face and neck the channel roughly follows the passage of the mouth, pharynx and oesophagus, but at the level of the clavicle it does something interesting – it moves dramatically away from the neck to the middle of the clavicle to a point known as *Que Pen* (Empty Basin) ST-12.

Western doctors should know this point well: it is the exact site of Virchov's node, a *pathognomonic* (diagnostic) site for lymph node spread in stomach cancer (on the left side; on the right side it is often from oesophagus or lung cancer). For Western doctors the cancer spreads here because of the lymphatic drainage, for Eastern because of the flow of pathological Qi.

Both occur in the fascia and so there is really little dispute between East and West; in fact Western medicine should really give Chinese medicine some credit and call this Que Pen's node.

Yang   From *Que Pen* ST-12 the channel descends downwards. It passes through the nipple and then continues down to the abdomen. At the abdomen it veers towards the midline before continuing down along the *rectus abdomini* muscle.

The relationship between the nipple and Gut channel is more intimate than chance. In other mammals, for instance dogs, there is a chain of nipples and this chain follows the exact same trajectory as the Gut channel, moving inwards at the boundary of chest and abdomen. Rarely, some humans are born with accessory nipples (such as the fictional character Scaramanga in the Bond film *The Man with the Golden Gun*) and these nipples are most commonly found along the exact same line as the Gut channel.

James Bond's nipple was a poor fake, though, being inside from the nipple, not down. Bond was lucky that his enemies didn't have a degree in embryology, otherwise his fake nipple could have come, quite literally, unstuck.

The nipple itself behaves like a gut to the infant, being the origin of fluids and having already rotted and ripened grain to provide a perfect food: breast milk. In fact, the milk from the nipples is so perfect that sometimes breast-fed infants pass almost no stools. In poetic language the nipple is the connection between mother's stomach and baby, but maybe it is in fascial anatomy too?

As the body forms, the gut develops and the body wall envelops the contents. Just like the filling from a Swiss roll squeezing out, there will be a fascial line of connection to the layers of the gut. This line might be simple, or more complex.

Charles Darwin thought that mammary glands emerged from sweat glands that were more nutritious than normal, but evolutionary biologists are still not sure how they developed. I'm going to hazard a guess…

The Gut channel (nipple line) of Chinese medicine represents a fascial plane that communicates with the layers of the gut. At some point in evolution some animals had a defective channel; fluid rich in fat and nutrients from the gut poured out from this line and their offspring took advantage. Over time this characteristic was selected and the nipples became more prominent…mammals emerged.

The kind of fluid that gets squeezed out between fascia is called *Yang*
lymph, and breast milk is very similar to this as it contains no
cells and is high in fat. Over time, evolution made breasts, but at
first – just as Charles Darwin intimated – it may have just been a
leaky fascial plane.

Given that there's little in the way of explanation of how
mammary glands evolved, and the Chinese state this is the Gut
channel, I'm willing to bet this is right!

The actual Gut channel is easy to explain from *Que Pen* ST-12
to the leg. It follows a plane in the body created by the internal
mammary artery! This cuts inwards at the junction of ribs and
abdomen (just as the Gut channel does) to form the superior
epigastric artery. This then connects with the inferior epigastric
artery before joining the external iliac artery.

This is a very unusual thing for arteries to do in the body
– connect together rather than gradually disperse – which is
why anatomists give it a special name (in Greek, of course) – an
anastomosis. As a result of this anastomosis there is a single fascial
connection from *Que Pen* ST-12 to the leg, just as Acupuncture
theory teaches.

It is important to understand that the arteries are not the Gut
channel – rather, they mark it out. Qi is the commander of Blood:
where Qi goes, Blood will follow. The same is true here – the Qi is
directing the blood to flow in this way.

The external iliac artery sits in the same plane as TaiYin
(anterior pararenal), hence the connection between the Gut and
Spleen channels.

The artery follows the line of the Gut channel perfectly –
cutting inwards under the ribs. It also moves up the middle of
the (underside of the) rectus muscle, just as the Gut channel does.

At the leg the Gut channel does something weird: it crosses
over the Spleen channel. Acupuncture channels shouldn't do this
– if they cross over it means that the information, the Qi, crosses
over too and that could cause confusion. This may have something
to do with how the gut itself is constantly moving between JueYin
and TaiYin.

Yang   The important thing to understand about the Acupuncture channels is that they are not real. By that I do not mean that they do not exist, but that the delineation of the channels is an artificial construct. When man maps the oceans or great rivers of the continents he creates artificial boundaries where none really exist. The Indian Ocean is defined by the contours of Africa and Asia before it turns into the Atlantic Ocean on its westward flank and the Southern Ocean on its the eastern. In reality there is only one body of water but the distinction is useful. In the same way the division of rivers into tributaries is arbitrary but useful. The Acupuncture channels are no different: they are real but the naming of them is an artificial construct in order to achieve some form of order out of the apparent chaos.

When the Spleen and Gut channels 'cross over' it means that in reality they are one channel with two different aspects – a Yin and a Yang if you like.

The Gut Channel…Again

The Leg YangMing has already been covered – the Gut channel.

The Large Intestine channel starts at the nose where it can be seen as a continuation of the Gut channel and then (uniquely) crosses the midline and travels down the neck of the opposite side. From here it goes to *Que Pen* (Empty Basin) ST-12 where it re-meets the Gut channel and then separates to flow down in the fascial planes of the arm, and forearm.

This channel is the arm equivalent of the Gut channel, which is why the Chinese pair them and call them Arm and Leg YangMing. They are really just two aspects of the same channel, one going to the arm and the other to the leg.

Emergency case report   *Yang*

I have often found the points on the Arm TaiYang (Large Intestine) channel to be useful for neck pain (especially *He Gu*, LI-4), and also for toothache (*Pian Li* LI-6). The Stomach channel can be used for Bell's palsy and also for shoulder problems (see Dr Wang Ju-Yi's book).[1]

30

ShaoYang (Lesser Yang)

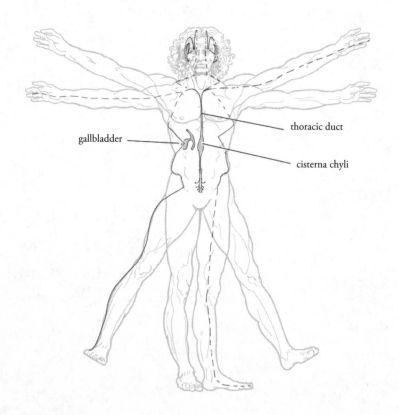

gallbladder

thoracic duct

cisterna chyli

The Lymph Channel   *Yang*

In Chinese parlance, to have good Gallbladder means to show determination to follow things through, to remain upright, to have courage. Searching for a logic behind the Gallbladder channel has, appropriately enough, been a test of my gallbladder organ.

When I started this book I didn't realise where it was going to go. I knew there was an explanation for Acupuncture's effects, and that the channels were real entities in the fascia, but what I honestly did not expect was such perfect correlation between East and West. How could the Bladder channel, for example, ever make any sense?

The Gallbladder channel was even more difficult to understand, though. It's the strangest channel. Yang channels are on the outside in the fascia of muscles – so how does it find its way inside to wrap around the gallbladder, which is resolutely intra-peritoneal?

The Gallbladder is also very intimate with the actual fascia and tendons (which are condensed fascia): its channel runs in the *temporalis* fascia and down the only muscle with fascia in its name – the *tensor fascia latae* in the leg; the Gallbladder point *Yang Ling Quan* (Yang Mound Spring) GB-34 is the pre-eminent point in the body to relax tendons, and the Gallbladder controls the Qi of tendons, keeping them supple. Why does the Gallbladder have such strong ties to the fascia?

The physical gallbladder sits next to the liver in the JueYin, the deepest Yin level in the body. How does the channel get in there?

Jue doesn't really mean deepest, though. Jue is drawn as a mountain with an opening in its side. Jue means 'reverting' and the reverting that this channel talks about is Yin reverting to Yang.

When the layers of the bowel are drawn, they resemble the six layers of the body; only JueYin is on the outside of the bowel. This is because the bowel is *Yang within Yin*.

JueYin is the ultimate Yin level and what it has to do is revert back to Yang. This is basic Yin/Yang theory: excessive Yin will

Yang convert to Yang. JueYin takes the rich and nutritious fluid and Qi and moves it back into…the lymph of ShaoYang.

In Western medicine it is accepted that the fluid in the peritoneum actually travels in a circuit, starting at the liver, working its way around the bowel, dipping into the pelvis where it communicates with the outside through the fallopian tubes and then going back to end under the liver. Here at the liver there is an opening between the towering walls of the liver and the diaphragm. This fluid is absorbed into the lymph.

This is the actual JueYin.

Western medicine calls it the *submesothelial lymphatics* in the *paracolic gutter*. Once again, JueYin is easier to say!

The fluid from this gets absorbed into the collection of lymph nodes called the *cisterna chyli*…which sit directly below the gallbladder. *Cisterna* is Latin for a cavity and *chyli* means fat suspension: this is a big cavity in the body containing a milky fatty suspension. This fluid doesn't just contain what the peritoneum produced, it also contains a lot of the fats that have been absorbed into the lymph of the gut.

The fats in the body have a special circulation – they don't get absorbed into the blood from the gut; instead they go into the lymphatics in the form of *chylomicrons* (Latin for 'little fatty balls'). After a very fatty meal the liquid in this cavity would look like milk!

The *cisterna chyli* is the Grand Central Station of the body's lymphatics, and the gallbladder sits right on top of it.

Of course, it goes without saying that the fluid around the gallbladder drains straight into the *cisterna chyli*: it would be improper to suggest otherwise (this is a Chinese medicine joke – ha, ha).

The relation between gallbladder and lymph isn't just from proximity – it is also functional! The gallbladder is responsible for absorbing fats correctly: it stores *gall*, which it releases to ensure fat is absorbed into the lymph properly. Gall breaks the fats down. It is a subtle connection that means that when there is too much fat the gallbladder can respond.

In this way the gallbladder is the organ of lymph and of fat and in the six layers of the body this works perfectly because the lymph glands sit directly behind the aorta (ShaoYin channel).

Yang

This links the gallbladder to fat, to lymph, and so through the lymphatic channels up into the shoulder and down into the pelvis to 'emerge on the sacrum' (as Deadman describes it).[1] In fact, it also provides an explanation for another type of referred pain experienced by people with gallbladder disease, or sometimes people who get blood near this area (such as in ruptured ectopic pregnancies). This pain goes to the shoulder tip.

Doctors have used 'confused brain theory' to explain this away with nerves (again the poor phrenic nerve gets the blame), but a better explanation is that it is following the fascial pathways of the lymphatic vessels into the *thoracic duct*.

Blood, pus or even air (!) from keyhole surgery can be very irritating and this pain would travel along the lymphatic system. From here the pathological Qi travels upwards (along with the flow of the thoracic duct) to finally irritate the nerves where it drains into the *subclavian* veins. These veins are deep in the shoulder and would account for the pain being felt in the shoulder.

How does this link in with tendons and fascia, though? Chinese medicine is explicit about the Gallbladder being responsible for providing the Qi for tendons (tendons are like highly condensed fascia). Furthermore, many Gallbladder points are found in areas of high concentration of fascia.

Fat problems (high cholesterol) and tendon problems are well linked; in fact people who have ruptured tendons should be screened for cholesterol problems![2] High cholesterol is an example of fat that isn't under control, a role that the gallbladder is critical in: thus the Chinese link between the Gallbladder and supple tendons actually makes sense!

Cholesterol in some way can make fascia and tendons tangle up on themselves, and can even create lumps in them called *xanthomas*. All the Yang organs are in fact *channels* and the Gallbladder is no exception: its close relationship to tendons and fascia is because these are bloodless and so are nourished with lymph. The tiny

Yang   channels in these structures carrying lymph are controlled by the Gallbladder function of keeping the lymph clean.

The Gallbladder channel is the channel of lymph – the lymphatic system.

The Channel of Tao

At the very beginning of this book I talk about God…quite a lot!

I don't believe in God, though; I believe in the Tao (or Dao).

What is the Tao? It is best described in the first lines of the 2600-year-old classic of philosophy, the *Tao Te Ching*:

The Tao that can be described is not the Tao.

What this means is the moment you describe it, you limit it and then by the very nature of the Tao you are no longer quite describing it.

It is like a de-anthropomorphisized God, with the same omniscience but none of the social baggage. The laws of science that we describe are really (to paraphrase Stephen Hawking) the mind of the Tao. The Tao is also translated as 'the way'; as in, the way in which one goes on a journey. The philosophy of Taoism is the spiritual application of this to life.*

Our incredible development from single cell to complex, beautiful, amazing creatures is an example of the Tao's way. If you prefer to use 'God' you can; it really is semantics.

And in the body this energy flows in the fascia, and the channel of the fascial spaces is the Triple Burner channel. It flows on from

---

*   For a truly outstanding enunciation of the ways of Taoism read *The Tao of Pooh* by Benjamin Hoff.[3]

the lymph of the Gallbladder channel as the *lymphatic system* of *Yang*
the upper body.

The lymph lives in the fascia, and so the Triple Burner is the
channel of fascia itself. Using points on this influences how the
fascia physically opens up or closes.

So we are back full circle, back to fascia, back to that mysterious
substance that probably meant nothing to you when you first
opened this book.

Now we understand differently. Fascia is everywhere –
controlling everything; forming our body; channelling Qi; keeping
everything in order. And the Triple Burner is the channel of fascia
– God's channel; the channel of the Tao.

Emergency case report

Headaches often respond to massage of the Gallbladder channel.
Headaches occur in the fascia (predominantly – see Appendix 3)
and massage of the Gallbladder channel aids the flow of lymph
in the fascia and thus helps release this tension. I find the
poetically named *Zu Lin Qi* (Foot Overlooking Tears) GB-41
to be particularly useful in Gallbladder-type headaches. Often it
will release tears and with them the emotional frustration that
lies behind many headaches. I normally pair it with points on the
Triple Burner channel, such as *Wai Guan* (Outer Frontier Gate)
TB-5.

Basic knowledge of acupressure and massage can do enormous
things for patients in Emergency Departments and hospitals. In
Chinese medicine you are not considered a *ripe* practitioner until
you are at least 60, so even I still have a long way to go (I hope).
Despite that, many of my patients benefit from simple techniques

that reduce pain, increase mobility, and sometimes even 'cure' their conditions. Anyone can learn these techniques.

It is my sincere hope that more and more Western practitioners will start using Acupressure/puncture, raising the standard of care for their patients. As the principles of Acupuncture become accepted and understood, Acupuncture will resume its rightful place – as an integral first-line treatment for the sick patient.

Epilogue

One of the leading websites on Evidence Based Medicine – Bandolier (www.medicine.ox.ac.uk/bandolier) – used to have this as its tagline:

Know what you are measuring.

It was a pertinent way of pointing out the problem of bias and confounding factors in a trial – bias will wreck trials as surely as a train will wreck a car left on its line. If you know what you are measuring then you will know if there is any bias or any confounding factors present.

The gold standard of trials is the double-blind randomised controlled trial (DBRCT). The trial eliminates two of the most important sources of error in clinical trials: observer bias and placebo effect. This kind of trial is uniquely appropriate for pharmaceuticals where a placebo and trial pill can be interchanged with complete anonymity. The trials have revolutionised medical care with pharmaceuticals and destroyed many misconceptions about what works in medicine.

Beyond the DBRCT we have to use other, less 'controlled', trials. Trials of sunscreen, for instance, have always been cohort studies where populations who use and don't use sunscreen are compared. Interestingly the evidence is contrary to what you might have thought you knew – the more sunscreen you use, the more skin cancer you get. Researchers tried to remove the confounding issue in this – that the more sunscreen you use, the more sun exposure you tend to have – but never really got rid of the sunscreen and skin cancer association. At the heart of these studies lies the single incontrovertible rule: if the sun is going to burn you then stay out of it.

Another type of trial that can be done is an interventionist trial. These trials tend to have unintended consequences. When well-meaning campaigners tried to mandate cycle helmet use for all they ended up with fewer people cycling. In an increasingly obese population such an effect is, laughably, tragic.

Medical researchers have tried to apply the rules of double-blind randomised control trials to Acupuncture. They have created sham needles and sham points. They have 'blinded' patients and tried to make the entire process standardised. They are forgetting one thing though: do *they* know what they are measuring?

Chinese medicine and Acupuncture are holistic; in other words a symptom only has meaning when taken in context of the whole. Western medicine tends to be reductionist: if you are breathless and get a diagnosis of asthma then the treatment will be the same regardless of who you are. In Chinese medicine the following can cause what would be considered to be asthma:

- Liver Qi stagnation invading Lungs.

- Lung Qi deficiency.

- Spleen Qi deficiency causing Phlegm in the Lungs.

- Kidney Qi not holding Lung Qi.

I have seen all these conditions in the Emergency Department and I would treat them all the same way: corticosteroids, nebulised B-agonists, IV fluids, magnesium and, in extremis, adrenaline. The Chinese diagnosis is much different, though, and depends on the patient. Some patients are asthmatic purely because of their damp, mouldy houses; some because they have unresolved issues of grief; and some because they have a liver which isn't working properly.

I have helped patients with acupressure – the point *Kong Zui* (Collection Hole) LU-6 is particularly helpful at moving Lung Qi and resolving stagnation – but every patient remains resolutely different. How do you standardise this? You can't!

Not only that, but you can't standardise the practitioner either – some practitioners are no good, some are geniuses. Throw six practitioners into a trial and what you will get is six different effects into one.

What are Acupuncture trials measuring exactly?

First, we have to ask if the treatment is 'standardised'. If it is then it is no longer Chinese medicine, unless of course you have gone to the trouble of 'standardising' the patients too.

Presuming that the treatments are not standardised then have you used sham points? There are no such things as 'sham points': the points are places in the connective tissue that conduct Qi, but connective tissue, and hence Qi, is everywhere! When a large German trial showed that Acupuncture was more effective than physiotherapy in chronic back pain, the detractors cried loudest:

'But the sham Acupuncture worked almost as well!'

Well, that's because it's still Acupuncture, isn't it?!

Sham points don't exist – there are strong points and weak points. What you are measuring with 'sham Acupuncture' is more like 'non-specific Acupuncture'. Whether this is better than Acupuncture is still a valid question to ask, but, in the words of Bandolier, you have to know what you are measuring.

Not only are there no 'sham points', but there are also good Acupuncturists and bad Acupuncturists. When studying with the legendary Dr Wang Ju-Yi I noticed his points never bled. When he described how Acupuncture occurs in the spaces in the tissue he said:

'You may have noticed that my points rarely bleed – that is because I am getting the spaces in the tissues where there are no blood vessels.'

I had never heard this before in three and a half years of Acupuncture school but it immediately made sense and it made me wonder how deeply the concepts of Acupuncture had been thought about in the modern world. Dr Wang Ju-Yi was the first 'scientific' Acupuncturist I had met, and his teachings are the impetus for this book.

One of my profound hopes is that this book will help to crystallise your thoughts on what exactly we are doing with Acupuncture. There is a science of Acupuncture, but in order to discover it we need to be scientific. Too many Acupuncturists are woolly minded and unquestioning, and too many doctors are pig-headed and arrogant. Ignoring 5000 years of medical tradition and healing because you don't understand it is not being scientific, it is being stupid and ignorant. Likewise, blindly following 5000 years of tradition because you don't have a curious and sceptical mind is bound to send you up a blind alley.

What Dr Wang Ju-Yi did was quite remarkable. He took his clinical experience and developed a new system of Acupuncture based on channel palpation and finding the spaces in the body. But it wasn't new! As an avid reader of the classics he eventually found that the *NeiJing SuWen* (remember that written Chinese is difficult for Chinese too!) stated this about Acupuncture all along. He was relieved that this was the case, for within his professional circle there is only truth if it is to be found in the classics. This attitude still persists today and it is backwards: Acupuncturists need to embrace anatomy and physiology, stem cells and genetics, bio-energy and electromagnetism, but we need to do it with intelligence. The classics were written to pass down information through turbulent primitive times. It is testament to their power and truth how well they have succeeded.

Now we must build on them...

APPENDIX 1

HOW CANCER MOVES

Cancer is defined by two factors. First, it is uncontrolled multiplication of cells and, second, these cells invade other tissues. The latter point is critical: tumours that do not invade are called benign tumours and will not kill you. They can grow to considerable size, like lipomas or fibroids, but they never cross fascial boundaries – if they did they would be considered to be malignant. Cancer itself is considered to spread in one of three ways and medics often describe this as the TNM system.

The 'T' stands for tumour and is a measure of how locally invasive the original cancer is. Cancer spreads into the tissue forming the organ where it grew from, but this in itself rarely causes problems. Few cancers cause problems during this stage because the cancer is just a lump. This is the basis of why we need screening programmes: we know that if we catch cancer before it has spread through the fascia of its organ we have a much better chance of curing it. The problem is that it rarely causes symptoms at this stage. When the cancer has grown into surrounding organs then removing it is far more difficult. The highest and worst stage in this system is where it invades through its own fascia.

'N' stands for (lymph) nodes. Lymph nodes are the police stations of the fascia. All of the fluid that ends up between the cells either gets absorbed back into the blood or gets squeezed into the lymphatic system through tiny lymphatic capillaries. Lymph nodes live in the fascia; you don't find them in tissues, you find them in the space between tissues and organs. The lymphatic system is ultra-important in controlling both microbes and cancer cells, as they filter all this fluid and decide what can go through and what needs to be destroyed. This is why lymph nodes get inflamed when bacterial infection starts spreading beyond the tissue it started in. It is also why cancer spreads to lymph nodes.

Examples of cancer spreading through nodes include breast cancer spreading to lymph glands under the armpit, stomach and lung cancer to lymph glands above the clavicle, and testicular cancer to lymph glands in the groin. All of these glands sit in the fascial planes.

'M' stands for metastasis. These are spots of cancer that have spread a long way away. To do this cancer often uses the blood. Blood is considered to be a 'connective tissue', because its cells connect things using plasma as its matrix. Normally cells do not invade into the blood, since most of the blood in the body is partitioned off by the use of *tight junctions* that prevent all but the smallest molecules from crossing. Of course, healthy cells have no desire to enter into the blood and if they do this accidentally then they get filtered out by the spleen. Gap junctions are missing in the liver and spleen, which may partially explain why cancer so often spreads to these organs. Blood isn't delineated by fascia: to perform its function of nourishment and protection it needs to get close to tissues, and fascia by its nature prevents this.

The spread of cancer through blood does not involve fascia, but this is not at odds with Acupuncture theory. In fact cancer is often seen as 'congealed blood' in Chinese medicine – an awareness that cancer results in abnormal blood. In the 'T' and the 'N' of the TNM system fascia is, however, very important in movement.

It shouldn't really come as a surprise that fascia is so involved in cancer prognosis. Fascia delineates tissue, it tells things where they should be, and cells that ignore this are by their nature nasty.

YIN AND YANG

In order to understand Chinese medicine you must also understand the basis of Chinese philosophical thought. Yin and Yang are at the heart of Chinese medicine and there is no better way to explain the philosophy of Yin and Yang than through the *Taijitu* (the Supreme Ultimate), better known as the Yin/Yang symbol.

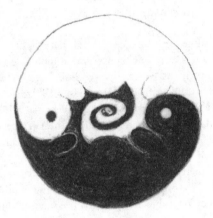

The symbol contains a number of features that explain the simple themes of Yin/Yang philosophy:

- *Yin and Yang form a whole.* They cannot exist without each other, but together they complete each other. They are complementary but opposite, like night and day.
- *Yin and Yang are constantly moving, and transforming into each other.* This is represented by the swirling nature of the Supreme Ultimate.
- *Excessive Yin turns into Yang and vice versa.* This is represented by the smaller dots within the swirls of black and white.

Yin and Yang are used to describe the nature of everything in the heavens and on Earth. It is a powerful philosophical model and one that can always be applied to the workings of nature. For instance, the day emerges from the night, becomes brighter and then at its zenith starts forming the night again. If there is too much heat then storm clouds will be created and cool the day down again: excessive Yang creating Yin. In society if capitalists (Yang) get too rich then the majority of workers (Yin) will rise up and overthrow them.

In the body we also have Yin and Yang, which science describes in terms of homeostasis, or normalcy. Blood pressures and temperatures can be too high (Yang) or low (Yin), blood too acid or alkali, muscles too tight (Yang) or too loose (Yin). Chinese medicine takes this a step further by describing the organs themselves in terms of Yin and Yang.

The Yin organs resemble Yin, the feminine, earthly, solid, watery, dark aspect of the duality. These organs are more solid, nourishing, static and store vital purified substances. They are also vital: we cannot live without these organs. The Yin organs are Kidney, Pancreas and Spleen, Liver, Lung and Heart. The latter two, an observant reader may note, can be considered to be hollow as well. For this reason, and the fact that they are also at the upper (Yang) part of the body, they are considered to be the most Yang of the Yin organs.

Yang is masculine, heavenly, ephemeral, fiery, light – all the opposites of Yin. Yang organs are hollow, active and responsible for moving stuff. In contrast to Yin organs we can live without one or two of these. The Yang organs, such as the Stomach, Intestines, Gallbladder and Bladder, are responsible for moving and extracting substances. To achieve this they are hollow organs and are constantly moving. Like the Yin organs there is further subdivision – the Gallbladder is considered more Yin than the Bladder, for instance.

Furthermore, there are the extraordinary organs. These are extraordinary because they are hollow organs that are filled with useful purified substances. For this reason they resemble Yang organs in structure, but Yin organs in function. They include the brain, uterus, bone marrow and Gallbladder – the last both extraordinary and Yang.

The brain has very little significance in Chinese medicine, since most of its functions are ascribed to other organs. In our brain-centric modern world this can seem perverse, but, as we have seen, the brain chemicals that help us think are also found in the organs. The brain is seen to govern in Chinese medicine, a role that is analogous to a computer. The Chinese called it the *peculiar organ* which, given the ongoing mystery of how it works, is still a good description of it to this day.

The philosophy of Yin and Yang is infinitely flexible, Yang within Yin within Yang *ad infinitum*. The day may be Yang, but the evening is more Yin than the morning as people are getting ready to rest rather than get busy. As the evening wears on it turns not more Yin but more Yang as people get up and party.

In the body, Yin/Yang philosophy is merely a description. The Taoists define the Tao as:

The Tao that can be described is not the Tao.

This description in terms of Yin and Yang cannot be followed too closely, however. For example, the Heart appears to be Yang in nature as it moves, is hollow, and houses the *Shen* – the Chinese word for the ephemeral spiritual, Yang-like, nature of ourselves. Yet, it is a Yin organ because it stores and moves our vital blood. It is the most Yang of the Yin organs.

The classification of these organs may be different but all of them have a parallel in Western medicine and once we have overcome problems of translation (philosophical, cultural and linguistic) they mainly agree on the physiology. However, Western medicine has no concept of what is called the Triple Burner.

'REFERRED' OR 'RADIATING' PAIN

One of the most perplexing questions that we are faced with is why heart attack pain goes to different places in different people, and specifically why it goes to the neck, jaw and arm.

It should be noted that the description of heart attack pain going along fascial pathways is at odds with the Western medical viewpoint on why heart pain is felt in the arm and neck. Put simply, the Western viewpoint is that the brain is too dumb to know its arse from its elbow (or in this case its heart from its elbow). Studies show this just isn't true, though – the brain does know the difference. Scientists have even coined a new word to describe the brain's awareness of the organs – interoception.[1]

The Western viewpoint of 'referred pain' goes somewhat like this. Different nerves supply different parts of the body, but if those nerves plug into the same part of the spinal cord then the brain thinks they're from the same place. It is like having two electrical devices connected to the same meter – you don't know one which is running.

In the case of a heart attack it is thought that pain in the heart irritates the diaphragm and the pericardium registers and transmits pain signals. These pain signals go to the level of the third to fifth cervical nerve roots in the spinal cord. The skin supplied by these roots is over the neck and upper arm, chest wall and arm, and so the brain, not knowing which the pain is from, registers it in the wrong place or both.

Instead of 'confused brain theory', why not a theory of fascial propagation? If the pain is travelling down the fascia then it will be doing this in the same way that electricity radiates down through copper wires or along water. We know the fluid between the fascia conducts electricity.

Nerves innervate fascia and nerves also choose to travel in fascia so the connection between the two is strong. Instead of 'confused brain', why can't the pain be actually radiating along the fascial planes through the network of nerves? The stronger the pain and the more intense the electrical signal, the stronger the radiation will be. This is consistent with what the studies show. Local anaesthetic in the area in these cases should abolish the referred pain stimulus. Very few studies have been done on this but at least one has showed that this is the case.[2]

There are three types of referred pain: somatic (or organ pain), radiculopathy (or nerve damage pain) and muscular referred pain.

Radiculopathic pain is where a nerve gets damaged and sends aberrant messages to the brain. The brain here is truly being fooled because the pain nerves that supply distal parts of the body are being triggered at a place where nature never intended to trigger them. This pain is common in slipped discs and other spinal problems. The nerve itself is enclosed in its own fascia and it is along this fascia that the Qi travels. There is no contradiction between this and the fascial theory of referred pain as radiculopathic pain is a special type – injured nerve pain.

Muscular fascial pain moves along between the muscles. Here, when muscles become tight they tangle their fascial envelopes. The body is a web and once any part moves the whole web has to readjust. This is known as the body *tensegrity* system. To most people who work on the body (e.g. masseurs/physios) as opposed to with the body (e.g. doctors) this will seem self-evident. Depending on which muscles are tight, various planes of the body readjust and it does this along fairly predictable lines. These lines have been described as the (especially the Yang) Acupuncture channels of Chinese medicine.

Finally we have somatic radiating pain. Somatic means 'body' but in this sense it is used to refer to 'internal organ'.

The most well-known example of referred pain is the heart itself. Instead of 'confused brain theory', this can be seen as pain radiating along the pathways of the major arteries into the face and arm.

Oesophageal referred pain goes up to the throat and down into the stomach – these are the fascial planes of the gut.

Appendix pain begins at the middle of the abdomen when only the fascia surrounding the appendix is stretched. Despite the appendix being in the bottom right-hand corner of our bellies, the fascial connection runs via the mesentery to the midline of the back around the level of the umbilicus. This is where the pain of appendicitis classically (i.e. 10–15% of the time) starts. Then, when it has irritated the fascia on the wall of the abdomen, it moves there.

Pelvic pain often refers into the inner thighs, through the Kidney channel/obturator canal – the only exit of the pelvis into the legs.

Rectal pain refers down the fascia into the anus.

Bladder pain moves down the fascia of the urethra into the tip of the penis, or the fascia into the testicles.

No one is quite sure what causes ice cream headaches, but one theory states they are caused by dilation of the arteries that go into the brain. When you eat something very cold this can cause dilation of the arteries to the brain which pass through the nose (kind of). When they dilate it pulls on the *dura* fascia of the brain causing the characteristic pounding headache!

In a very similar way, anything that causes the arteries to dilate will give a headache, and migraines are one example.

Pancreatic pain radiates into the back – a reflection of its connections.

Ureteric pain follows the Middle-kidney to the testicles, whereas kidney pain stays true to its embryological origins and stays in the loin.

The Lungs aren't considered to radiate pain but that is because if they do it goes to the voice box and people make the connection anyway.

Bone pain stays true to its location until it breaks through the fascia of the bone, then it can radiate along the fascia of the muscle planes.

Blood vessel pain radiates along the blood vessels – when the aorta tears, patients actually describe it as a tearing sensation in their back upon which the aorta runs.

Facial pain moves along the planes of the pharyngeal arches from which they develop.

Gallbladder pain and free blood in the peritoneum causes pain to radiate up the *cisterna chyli* into the subclavian veins and hence locates to the shoulder tip.

In fact, almost all radiation of pain can be described equally validly using fascia instead of 'confused brain theory'. The fascial Qi theory of pain referral predicts the radiation of pain rather than retrospectively describing it as is necessary with a confused and idiotic brain.

Furthermore, no brain idiocy needs to be assumed, as the brain is accurately registering where it feels the pain; it is the pain in the form of pathological elecQicity that is moving. The pathological elecQicity moves down the fascial planes, or Acupuncture channels as they are known, and it does this because the pain is a form of aberrant electrical activity that moves along the fascial planes. As it does this it causes further pain to develop.

Fascia is actually far more sensitive to pain than any of the organs.

Headaches are not caused by pain in the brain – the brain has no pain receptors and can be operated on when the patient is awake – rather, they are caused by fascial irritation.

Most of the gut transmits pain only when the fascia is stretched, hence the vague nature of abdominal cramping/bloating/ distending feeling that people often complain of.

Liver and spleen are insensitive to pain until their fascia become involved.

Kidney tumours create only a vague ache (caused by stretching of the fascia) until they erode through it.

Western medicine accepts that heart pain is felt in the fascia (pericardium), not in the muscle.

The terrible pain of cancer only begins once fascia is involved; prior to this cancer is almost certainly painless (which is the big problem in catching it early).

In fact, what is so remarkable when you look at somatic (organ) pain is that it really doesn't exist. Hardly any of the organs actually have any pain receptors. This is why you can grow cancers, poison your liver and get emphysema without ever knowing about it.

The idea that organ pain is confused by the brain is nonsensical since no one has ever felt liver pain – there is only liver capsule (fascia) pain; brain tumours only cause pain when the dura matter (fascia) is stretched; and emphysema is painful when the lungs get so dry that the lung pleura (fascia) can't glide anymore (pleurisy).

The fascial Qi theory of radiation of pain not only beautifully describes pain radiation but it fits perfectly in with Acupuncture theory. Is it possible that Western medicine has made one of the biggest medical blunders of all time in missing this connection? Fascial Qi theory would predict that you could affect this pain by modulating the flow of elecQicity in the fascia, and pain relief is Acupuncture's greatest success. Three thousand years of medicine has been built on this one extraordinary property.

If this proves to be accepted I wish this to be known as the 'Daniel Keown Theory of Fascia and Acupuncture Pain'...

...only joking. It's just Acupuncture...innit!

ENDNOTES

Prologue

1. Illingworth, C.M. (1974) 'Trapped fingers and amputated finger tips in children.' *J. Pediatr. Surg. 9*, 6, 853–858.
2. Becker, R.O. and Seldon, G. (1985) *The Body Electric*. New York, NY: Morrow.

Chapter 3

1. Kumar, P. and Clark, M. (2012) *Clinical Medicine* (8th edition). Edinburgh: Saunders.
2. Longmore, M., Wilkinson, I. and Torok, E. (2001) *Oxford Handbook of Clinical Medicine* (5th Edition). Oxford: Oxford University Press.
3. Minary-Jolandan, M. and Yu, M.-F. (2009) 'Nanoscale characterization of isolated individual type I collagen fibrils: polarization and piezoelectricity.' *Nanotechnology 20*, 8.

Chapter 4

1. Berisio, R., Vitagliano, L., Mazzarella, L. and Zagari, A. (2002) 'Crystal structure of the collagen triple helix model [(Pro-Pro-Gly)10]3.' *Protein Sci. 11*, 2, 262–270.
2. Qin, Z., Gautieri, A., Nair, A.K., Inbar, H. and Buehler, M.J. (2012) 'Thickness of hydroxyapatite nanocrystal controls mechanical properties of the collagen-hydroxyapatite interface.' *Langmuir 28*, 4, 1982–1992. Available at www.ncbi.nlm.nih.gov/pubmed/22208454, accessed on 30 July 2013.
3. Minary-Jolandan, M. and Yu, M.-F. (2009) 'Nanoscale characterization of isolated individual type I collagen fibrils: polarization and piezoelectricity.' *Nanotechnology 20*, 8.

Chapter 5

1. Fernández, J.R., García-Aznar, J.M. and Martínez, R. (2012) 'Piezoelectricity could predict sites of formation/resorption in bone remodelling and modelling.' *J. Theor. Biol. 292*, 86–92.
2. Ferrier, J., Ross, S.M., Kanehisa J. and Aubin, J.E. (1986) 'Osteoclasts and osteoblasts migrate in opposite directions in response to a constant electrical field.' *J. Cell Physiol. 129*, 3, 283–288.
3. Hartig, M., Joos, U. and Wiesmann, H.P. (2000) 'Capacitively coupled electric fields accelerate proliferation of osteoblast-like primary cells and increase bone extracellular matrix formation in vitro.' *Eur. Biophys. J. 29*, 7, 499–506.
4. NASA (2011) *Space Bones*. Available at: http://science.nasa.gov/science-news/science-at-nasa/2001/ast01oct_1, accessed on 31 July 2013.
5. Panagiotidou, A. (July 2012) Personal discussions.
6. Tomaselli, V.P. and Shamos, M.H. (1974) 'Electrical properties of hydrated collagen. II. Semiconductor properties.' *Biopolymers 13*, 12, 2423–2434.
7. Becker, R.O. and Seldon, G. (1985) *The Body Electric*. New York, NY: Morrow.
8. Feng, J.F., Liu, J., Zhang, X.Z., Zhang, L. *et al.* (2012) 'Guided migration of neural stem cells derived from human embryonic stem cells by an electric field.' *Stem Cells 30*, 2, 349–355.

Chapter 6

1. Nugent-Head, A. (2011) *Demystifying Qi: Lecture 1*. Available at http://traditionalstudies.org/chinese-medicine/20-online-seminars-chinese-medicine/online-seminars/159-demystifying-qi, accessed on 31 July 2013.
2. Yang, J.-M. (2007) *Understanding Qigong* (DVD). Boston, MA: YMAA Publication Centre. Available at http://ymaa.com, accessed on 31 July 2013.

Chapter 7

1. Cohen, S. and Popp, F.A. (2003) 'Biophoton emission of the human body.' *Indian J. Exp. Biol. 41*, 5, 440–445.
2. Popp, F.A. (2003) 'Properties of biophotons and their theoretical implications.' *Indian J. Exp. Biol. 41*, 5, 391–402.
3. Takeda, M., Kobayashi, M., Takayama, M., Suzuki, S. *et al.* (2004) 'Biophoton detection as a novel technique for cancer imaging.' *Cancer Science 95*, 8, 656–661.
4. Jung, H.H., Woo, W.M., Yang, J.M., Choi, C. *et al.* (2003) 'Left-right asymmetry of biophoton emission from hemiparesis patients.' *Indian J. Exp. Biol. 4*, 5, 452–456.
5. Popp, F.A., Li, K.H., Mei, W.P., Galle, M. and Neurohr, R. (1988) 'Physical aspects of biophotons.' *Experientia 44*, 7, 576–585.

Chapter 8

1. Brimham, L., Eyre-Walker, A., Smith, N.H. and Smith, J.M. (2013) 'Mitochondrial Steve: paternal inheritance of mitochondria in humans.' *Trends in Ecology and Evolution.* Available at www.lifesci.sussex.ac.uk/home/Adam_Eyre-Walker/Website/Publications_files/BromhamTREE03.pdf, accessed on 1 August, 2013.
2. Carew, J.S. and Huang, P. (2002) 'Mitochondrial defects in cancer.' *Molecular Cancer 1*, 9.
3. Lane, N. (2005) *Power, Sex, Suicide: Mitochondria and the Meaning of Life.* Oxford: Oxford University Press.
4. Giraud-Guille, M.M., Besseau, L. and Martin, R. (2003) 'Liquid crystalline assemblies of collagen in bone and in vitro systems.' *J. Biomech. 36*, 10, 1571–1579.

Chapter 9

1. Grewal, P.K., Uchiyama, S., Ditto, D., Varki, N. *et al.* (2008) 'The Ashwell receptor mitigates the lethal coagulopathy of sepsis.' *Nature Medicine 14*, 6 648–655.

Chapter 11

1. Flachskampf, F.A., Gallasch, J., Gefeller, O., Gan, J. *et al.* (2007) 'Randomized trial of Acupuncture to lower blood pressure.' *Circulation 115*, 24, 3121–3129.
2. Lombardi, F., Belletti, S., Battezzati, P.M. and Lomuscio, A. (2012) 'Acupuncture for paroxysmal and persistent atrial fibrillation: an effective non-pharmacological tool?' *World J. Cardiol. 4*, 3, 60–65.
3. Lomuscio, A., Belletti, S., Battezzati, P.M. and Lombardi, F.J. (2011) 'Efficacy of Acupuncture in preventing atrial fibrillation recurrences after electrical cardioversion.' *Cardiovasc. Electrophysiol. 22*, 3, 241–247.
4. Martin, J., Donaldson, A.N.A., Villarroel, R., Parmar, M.K.B., Ernst, E. and Higginson, I.J. (2002) 'Efficacy of Acupuncture in asthma: systematic review and meta-analysis of published data from 11 randomised controlled trials.' *Eur. Respir. J. 20*, 4, 846–852.
5. Lee, A. and Fan, L.T. (2009) 'Stimulation of the wrist Acupuncture point P6 for preventing postoperative nausea and vomiting.' *Cochrane Database Syst. Rev. 15*, 2, CD003281.

6.   Ezzo, J., Streitberger, K. and Schneider, A. (2006) 'Cochrane systematic reviews examine P6 Acupuncture-point stimulation for nausea and vomiting.' *J. Altern. Complement. Med. 12*, 5, 489–495.

7.   Shang, C. (2001) 'Electrophysiology of growth control and acupuncture.' *Life Sciences 68*, 1333–1342.

Chapter 12

1.   Therapontos, C., Erskine, L., Gardner, E.R., Figg, W.D. and Vargesson, N. (2009) 'Thalidomide induces limb defects by preventing angiogenic outgrowth during early limb formation.' *P. Natl. Acad. Sci. USA 106*, 21, 8573–8578.

2.   Kaptchuk, T. (2000) *The Web That Has No Weaver.* New York, NY: McGraw-Hill. Available at http://disorders.free-books.biz/The-Web-That-Has-No-Weaver--Understanding-Chinese-Medicine-PDF-107.html, accessed on 2 August 2013.

3.   Albrecht-Buehler, G. (2012) 'Fractal genome sequences.' *Gene 498*, 1, 20–27.

4.   Blank, M. and Goodman, R. (2011) 'DNA is a fractal antenna in electromagnetic fields.' *Int. J. Radiat. Biol. 87*, 4, 409–415.

5.   Cattani, C. (2010) 'Fractals and hidden symmetries in DNA.' *Math. Probl. Eng.* Vol. 2010.

6.   Hahn, H.K., Georg, M. and Peitgen, H.-O. (2005) 'Fractal aspects of three-dimensional vascular constructive optimization.' In G.A. Losa and T.F. Nonnenmacher (eds) *Fractals in Biology and Medicine.* New York, NY: Springer.

7.   Kiselev, V.G., Hahn, K. and Auer, D.P. (2002) 'Is the brain cortex a fractal?' *Sonderforschungsbereich 386*, Discussion Paper 297. Available at http://epub.ub.uni-muenchen.de/1675, accessed on 2 August 2013.

8.   Narine, S. (1999) 'Fractal nature of fat crystal networks.' *Phys. Rev. E 59*, 1908–1920.

9.   Granek, R. (2011) 'Proteins as fractals: role of the hydrodynamic interaction.' *Phys. Rev. E 83*, 020902(R).

Chapter 13

1.   Biomimicry Institute (n.d.) *Fibonacci Sequence Optimizes Packing: Sunflowers.* Available at www.asknature.org/strategy/08ba894a508330861bac3ef1b574d804, accessed on 2 August 2013.

Chapter 15

1.   Bensky, D. and Gamble, A. (1986) *Chinese Herbal Medicine, Materia Medica.* Seattle, WA: Eastland Press.

2.   Chen, Y.J., Kuo, C.D., Chen, S.H., Chen, W.J. *et al.* (2007) 'Small-molecule synthetic compound norcantharidin reverses multi-drug resistance by regulating Sonic Hedgehog signaling in human breast cancer cells.' *Nat. Rev. Cancer 7*, 464–474.

3.   Pubmed search of 'sonic hedgehog' and 'cancer' taken on 1 September 2012.

4.   Screpanti, I., Modesti, A. and Gulino, S. (1993) 'Heterogeneity of thymic stromal cells and thymocyte differentiation: a cell culture approach.' *Journal of Cell Science 105*, 601–606.

5.   Potter, J. (2010) 'Models of carcinogenesis.' *Carcinogenesis 31*, 10, 1703–1709.

6.   Shang, C. (2007) 'Prospective tests on biological models of Acupuncture.' *Evid.Based Complemen. Alternat. Med. 6*, 1, 31–39.

7.   Mashanskii, V.F., Markov, I.V., Shpunt, V.K., Li, S.E. and Mirkin, A.S. (1983) 'Topography of the gap junctions in the human skin and their possible role in the non-neural signal transduction.' *Arkh. Anat. Gistol. Embriol. 84*, 53–60.

8.   Cui, H.-M. (1988) 'Meridian system – specialized embryonic epithelial conduction system.' *Shanghai J. Acupunct. 3*, 44–45.

9.   Fan, J.Y. (1990) 'The role of gap junctions in determining skin conductance and their possible relationship to Acupuncture points and meridians.' *Am. J. Acupunct. 18*, 163–170.

10. Wang, S.J., Omori, N., Li, F., Jin, G. *et al.* (2003) 'Functional improvement by electro-Acupuncture after transient middle cerebral artery occlusion in rats.' *Neurol. Res. 25*, 516–521.

11. Han, L., Da, C.D., Huang, Y.L. and Cheng, J.S. (2001) 'Influence of Acupuncture upon expressing levels of basic fibroblast growth factor in rat brain following focal cerebral ischemia – evaluated by time-resolved fluorescence immunoassay.' *Neurol. Res. 23*, 47–50.

12. Liang, X.B., Luo, Y., Liu, X.Y., Lu, J. *et al.* (2003) 'Electro-Acupuncture improves behavior and upregulates GDNF mRNA in MFB transected rats.' *Neuroreport 14*, 1177–1181.

13. Pan, B., Castro-Lopes, J.M., and Coimbra, A. (1996) 'Activation of anterior lobe corticotrophs by electroacupuncture or noxious stimulation in the anaesthetized rat, as shown by colocalization of Fos protein with ACTH and beta-endorphin and increased hormone release.' *Brain Res Bull. 40*, 175–182.

14. Lee, J.H. and Beitz, A.J. (1993) 'The distribution of brain-stem and spinal cord nuclei associated with different frequencies of electroacupuncture analgesia.' *Pain 52*, 11–28.

15. Stener-Victorin, E., Lundeberg, T., Waldenstrom, U., Manni, L. *et al.* (2000) 'Effects of electro-Acupuncture on nerve growth factor and ovarian morphology in rats with experimentally induced polycystic ovaries.' *Biol. Reprod. 63*, 1497–1503.

16. Bai, Y.H., Lim, S.C., Song, C.H., Bae, C.S. *et al.* (2004) 'Electro-Acupuncture reverses nerve growth factor abundance in experimental polycystic ovaries in the rat.' *Gynecol. Obstet. Invest. 57*, 80–85.

17. Liu, X., Shen, L., Wu, M., Wu, B. *et al.* (2004) 'Effects of Acupuncture on myelogenic osteoclastogenesis and IL-6 mRNA expression.' *J. Tradit. Chin. Med. 24*, 144–148.

Chapter 16

1. Dorfer, L., Moser, M., Bahr, F., Spindler, K. *et al.* (1999) 'A medical report from the stone age?' *Lancet 354*, 9183, 1023–1025.

Chapter 17

1. Kaptchuk, T. (2000) *The Web That Has No Weaver.* New York, NY: McGraw-Hill. Available at http://disorders.free-books.biz/The-Web-That-Has-No-Weaver--Understanding-Chinese-Medicine-PDF-107.html, accessed on 2 August 2013.

2. Ahn, A.C., Colbert, A.P., Anderson, B.J., Martinsen, Ø.G. *et al.* (2008) 'Electrical properties of Acupuncture points and meridians: a systematic review.' *Bioelectromagnetics 29*, 4, 245–256.

3. Langevin, H. and Yandrow, J. (2002) 'Relationship of Acupuncture points and meridians to connective tissue planes.' *Anat. Rec. 269*, 257–265.

4. Nuccitelli, R. (2003) 'Endogenous electric fields in embryos during development, regeneration and wound healing.' *Radiat. Prot. Dosimetry 106*, 4, 375–383.

5. Altizer, A.M. (2001) 'Endogenous electric current is associated with normal development of the vertebrate limb.' *Dev. Dyn. 22*, 4, 391–401.

6. Becker, R.O. and Seldon, G. (1985) *The Body Electric.* New York, NY: Morrow.

Chapter 19

1. Becker, D.L., David-LeClerc, C. and Warner, A.E. (1992) 'The relationship of gap junctions and compaction in the preimplantation mouse embryo.' *Development*, Supplement 'Gastrulation', 113–118.

2. Takaki, R. and Ueda, N. (2007) 'Analysis of spiral curves in traditional cultures.' *Forma 22*, 133–139.

Chapter 23

1.   Hershberger, S.L. (2001) 'Biological factors in the development of sexual orientation.' In A.R. D'Augelli and C.J. Patterson (eds) *Lesbian, Gay, and Bisexual Identities and Youth: Psychological Perspectives*. Oxford and New York: Oxford University Press.

Chapter 24

1.   Larsen, W.J. (1997) *Essentials of Human Embryology* (2nd Edition). New York, NY: Churchill Livingstone, p.86.

2.   Martinez-Morales, J.-R., Henrich, T., Ramialison, M. and Wittbrodt, J. (2007) 'New genes in the evolution of the neural crest differentiation program.' *Genome Biol. 8*, 3, R36.

3.   Clay, M.R. and Halloran, M.C. (2010) 'Control of neural crest cell behavior and migration: Insights from live imaging.' *Cell. Adh. Migr. 4*, 4, 586–594.

4.   Etchevers, H.C., Vincent, C. and Couly, G. (2001) 'Neural crest and pituitary development.' In R. Rappaport and S. Amselem (eds) *Hypothalmic-Pituitary Development: Genetic and Clinical Aspects*. Basel, Switzerland: Karger.

5.   Daily Mail (2013) 'Facial scans could reveal genetic disorders', 10 June. Available at www. dailymail.co.uk/health/article-480952/Facial-scans-reveal-genetic-disorders.html, accessed on 8 August 2013.

Chapter 25

1.   Seen on BBC4 programme: *Heart vs Mind: What Makes Us Human*. Broadcast 14 July 2012.

2.   De Vogli, R., Chandola, T. and Marmot, M.G. (2007) 'Negative aspects of close relationships and heart disease.' *Arch. Intern. Med. 167*, 18, 1951–1957.

3.   King, K.B. and Reis, H.T. (2012) 'Marriage and long-term survival after coronary artery bypass grafting.' *Health Psychol. 31*, 1, 55–62.

4.   Mostofsky, E., Maclure, M., Sherwood, J.B., Tofler, G.H., Muller, J.E. and Mittleman, M.A. (2012) 'Risk of acute myocardial infarction after the death of a significant person in one's life: the Determinants of Myocardial Infarction Onset Study.' *Circulation 125*, 3, 491–496.

5.   Pearsall, P., Schwartz, G. and Russek, L. (1999) 'Changes in heart transplant recipients that parallel the personalities of their donors.' *Integr. Med. 2*, 2/3, 65–72.

6.   NBC News (2008) 'Man with suicide victim's heart takes own life.' Available at: www. msnbc.msn.com/id/23984857/ns/us_news-life/t/man-suicide-victims-heart-takes-own-life/#. UD51gkRSRyI, accessed on 8 August 2013.

7.   The Washington Post (2007) 'His heart whirs anew.' Available at www.washingtonpost.com/ wp-dyn/content/article/2007/08/11/AR200708110 1390_4.html, accessed on 8 August 2013.

8.   Hall, B.K. (1999) *The Neural Crest in Development and Evolution*. New York, NY: Springer-Verlag.

9.   Deadman, P. and Al-Khafaji, M., with Baker, K. (2007) *A Manual of Acupuncture* (2nd edition). Hove: Journal of Chinese Medicine.

10. The Guardian (2010) 'Dozens killed by incorrectly placed Acupuncture needles.' Available at www.guardian.co.uk/science/2010/oct/18/dozens-killed-Acupuncture-needles, accessed on 8 August 2013.

11. Goldberg, S. (2010) *Clinical Anatomy Made Ridiculously Simple*. Medmaster.

12. Melamed, M.L., Blackwell, T., Neugarten, J., Arnsten, J.H. *et al.* (2011) 'A selective estrogen receptor modulator, is renoprotective: a post-hoc analysis.' *Kidney Int. 79*, 2, 241–249.

13. Yakushiji, Y., Nanri, Y., Hirotsu, T., Nishihara, M., Hara, M. and Nakajima, J. (2010) 'Marked cerebral atrophy is correlated with kidney dysfunction in nondisabled adults.' *Hypertens. Res. 33*, 12, 1232–1237.

14. Chun-yan Lu, C.-Y., Peng-qiu Min, P.-Q., and Bing Wu, B. (2012) 'CT evaluation of spontaneously ruptured renal angiomyolipomas with massive hemorrhage spreading into multi-retroperitoneal fascia and fascial spaces.' *Acta Radiol. Short Rep. 1*, 18.

15. O'Connell, A.M., Duddy, L., Lee, C. and Lee, M.J. (2007) 'CT of pelvic extraperitoneal spaces: an anatomical study in cadavers.' *Clin. Radiol. 62*, 5, 432–438.

Chapter 26

1. As with all embryology this is found in Larsen, W.J. (1997) *Essentials of Human Embryology* (2nd edition). New York, NY: Churchill Livingstone.

2. Personal discussion with Mr Asit Arora, Specialist Registrar in ENT and expert in robotic thyroid surgery. May 2013.

3. Hume, R. (2009) 'Thyroid hormone and lung development.' Available at www. hotthyroidology.com/editorial_82.html, accessed on 9 August 2013.

4. Deadman, P. and Al-Khafaji, M., with Baker, K. (2007) *A Manual of Acupuncture* (2nd edition). Hove: Journal of Chinese Medicine.

5. Watters, J.M., Sambasivan, C.N., Zink, K., Kremenevskiy, I. *et al.* (2010) 'Splenectomy leads to a persistent hypercoagulable state after trauma.' *Am. J. Surg. 199*, 5, 646–651.

6. Ley, E.J., Singer, M.B., Clond, M.A., Johnson, T. *et al.* (2012) 'Long-term effect of trauma splenectomy on blood glucose.' *J. Surg. Res. 177*, 1, 152–156.

7. Khan, Z.A.J. and Dikki, P.E. (2004) 'Return of a normal functioning spleen after traumatic splenectomy.' *J. R. Soc. Med. 97*, 8, 391–392.

8. Yagan, N., Auh, Y.H. and Fisher, A. (2009) 'Extension of air into the right perirenal space after duodenal perforation: CT findings.' *Radiology 250*, 740–748.

9. Plank, J.L., Mundell, N.A., Frist, A.Y., LeGrone, A.W. *et al.* (2011) 'Influence and timing of arrival of murine neural crest on pancreatic beta cell development and maturation.' *Dev Biol. 349*, 2, 321–330.

10. Asayesh, A., Sharpe, J., Watson, R.P., Hecksher-Sørensen, J. *et al.* (2006) 'Spleen versus pancreas: strict control of organ interrelationship revealed by analyses of Bapx1-/- mice.' *Genes Dev. 20*, 16, 2208–2213.

11. Unver Dogan, N., Uysal, I.I., Demirci, S., Dogan, K.H. and Kolcu, G. (2011) 'Accessory spleens at autopsy.' *Clin. Anat. 24*, 6, 757–762.

12. Paulmann, N., Grohmann, M., Voigt, J.-P., Bert, B., Vowinckel, J. *et al.* (2009) 'Intracellular serotonin modulates insulin secretion from pancreatic β-cells by protein serotonylation.' Available at www.plosbiology.org/article/info%3Adoi%2F10.1371%2Fjournal.pbio.1000229, accessed on 9 August 2013.

13. Khan, P.N., Nair, R.J., Olivares, J., Tingle, L.E. and Li, Z. (2009) 'Postsplenectomy reactive thrombocytosis.' *Proc. Bayl. Univ. Med. Cent. 22*, 1, 9–12.

14. Robinette, C.D. and Fraumeni, J. (1977) 'Splenectomy and subsequent mortality in veterans of the 1939–45 war.' *Lancet 310, 8029*, 127–129.

15. Goligorsky, M.S. (2007) 'Frontiers in nephrology: viewing the kidney through the heart – endothelial dysfunction in chronic kidney disease.' *J. Am. Soc. Nephrology 18*, 11, 2833–2835. Available at http://jasn.asnjournals.org/content/18/11/2833.full, accessed on 9 August 2013.

16. Lombard, M., Pastoret, P.P. and Moulin, A.M. (2007). 'A brief history of vaccines and vaccination.' *Rev. Sci. Tech. 26*, 1, 29–48.

17. Seeber, P. and Shander, A. (2012) *Basics of Blood Management*. Oxford: Wiley-Blackwell.

18. Simpson, L.O. and O'Neill, D.J. (2001) 'Red blood cell shapes in women with fibromyalgia and the implications for capillary blood flow and tissue function.' *J. Orthomol. Med. 16*, 4.

19. Ling, B.E. (2005) *Obsessive Compulsive Disorder Research*. New York, NY: Nova Science Publishers.

20. Ferguson, D., Doucette, S., Glass, K.C., Shapiro, S. *et al.* (2005) 'Association between suicide attempts and selective serotonin reuptake inhibitors: systematic review of randomised controlled trials.' *BMJ 330*, 7488, 396.

21. Winkler, T., Sharma, H.S., Stålberg, E., Olsson, Y. and Dey, P.K. (1995) 'Impairment of blood-brain barrier function by serotonin induces desynchronization of spontaneous cerebral cortical activity: experimental observations in the anaesthetized rat.' *Neuroscience 68*, 4, 1097–1104.

22. Abbott, N.J. (2000) 'Inflammatory mediators and modulation of blood-brain barrier permeability.' *Cell. Mol. Neurobiol. 20*, 2, 131–147.

23. Lotronex (2013) Available at www.lotronex.com, accessed on 9 August 2013.

24. Mellinkoff, S., Craddock, C., Frankland, M., Kendricks, F. and Greipel, M. (1962) 'Serotonin concentration in the spleen.' *Am. J. Dig. Dis. 7*, 347–355.

Chapter 27

1. Brulotte, S., Roy, L. and Larose, E. (2007) 'Congenital absence of the pericardium presenting as acute myocardial necrosis.' *Can. J. Cardiol. 23*, 11, 909–912.

2. Rubin, L, and Hudson, P. (1985) 'Epicardial versus parietal pericardial defibrillation.' *American Journal of Emergency Medicine 3*, 2, 160–164.

3. See, for example, Hameroff, S. (n.d.) 'Quantum computation in brain microtubules? The Penrose-Hameroff 'Orch OR' model of consciousness.' Available at www. quantumconsciousness.org/penrose-hameroff/quantumcomp utation.html, accessed on 10 August 2013.

4. Tzaphlidou, M. and Berillis, P. (2004) 'Effect of lithium administration on collagen and breaking pressure of the rat thoracic descending aorta.' *J. Trace Elem. Exp. Med. 17*, 3, 151–160.

5. Kounadi, E., Tzaphlidou, M., Fountos, G. and Glaros, D. (1995) 'An electron microscopic study of collagen fibril structure after lithium treatment – II. The effects of low lithium dose and short treatment on mouse skin collagen.' *Micron. 26*, 2, 113–120.

6. Larsen, W.J. (1997) *Essentials of Human Embryology* (2nd edition). New York, NY: Churchill Livingstone.

7. Maciocia, G. (2005) *The Foundations of Chinese Medicine* (2nd edition). New York, NY: Churchill Livingstone.

8. Roy, M. and Saha, E. (1982) *Anaesthesia*. Waltham, MA: Academic Press.

9. Lautt, W.W. and Greenway, C.V. (1976) 'Hepatic venous compliance and role of liver as a blood reservoir.' *Am. J. Physiol. 231*, 2, 292–295.

10. Lilja, B. and Lindell, S.E. (1961) 'Metabolism of 14C histamine in heart-lung-liver in cats.' *Br. J. Pharmacol. 16*, 2.

11. Drapanas, T., Adler, W. and Vang, J.O. (1965) 'Primary regulation of histamine metabolism by the liver.' *Ann. Surg. 161*, 3, 447–455.

12. Gittlen, S.D., Schulman, E.S. and Maddrey, W.C. (1990) 'Raised histamine concentrations in chronic cholestatic liver disease.' *Gut 31*, 1, 96–99.

13. Spahr, L., Coeytaux, A., Giostra, E., Hadengue, A. and Annoni, J.M. (2007) 'Histamine H1 blocker hydroxyzine improves sleep in patients with cirrhosis and minimal hepatic encephalopathy: a randomized controlled pilot trial.' *Am. J. Gastroenterol. 102*, 4, 744–753.

14. Sharma, S.C., Sheppard, B.L. and Bonnar, J. (1993) 'Uterine mast cell and histamine values in dysfunctional uterine bleeding.' *Inflammation Res. 38*, 3–4.

15. Livingstone, M. and Fraser, I.S. (2002) 'Mechanisms of abnormal uterine bleeding.' *Hum. Reprod. Update 8*, 66–67.

16. Maintz, L. and Novak, N. (2007) 'Histamine and histamine intolerance.' *Am. J. Clin. Nutr. 85*, 1185–1196.

17. Kasperska-Zajac, A., Brzoza, Z. and Rogala, B. (2008) 'Sex hormones and urticaria.' *J. Dermatol. Sci. 52*, 2, 79–86.

18. Cho, S., Kim, H.J., Oh, S.H., Park, C.O., Jung, J.Y. and Lee, K.H. (2010) 'The influence of pregnancy and menstruation on the deterioration of atopic dermatitis symptoms.' *Ann. Dermatol. 22*, 2, 180–185.

19. Joffe, H. and Hayes, F.J. (2008) 'Menstrual cycle dysfunction associated with neurologic and psychiatric disorders: their treatment in adolescents.' *Ann. NY Acad. Sci. 1135*, 219–229.

20. Herzog, A.G. (2006) 'Menstrual disorders in women with epilepsy.' *Neurology 66*, 6 (Suppl. 3), S23–28.

21. Schmidt, G., Ahrén, K., Brännström, M., Kannisto, P. *et al.* (1987) 'Histamine stimulates progesterone synthesis and cyclic adenosine 3',5'-monophosphate accumulation in isolated preovulatory rat follicles.' *Neuroendocrinology 46*, 1, 69–74.

22. Zierau, O., Zenclussen, A. and Jensen, F. (2012) 'Role of female sex hormones, estradiol and progesterone, in mast cell behavior.' *Front. Immunol. 19*, 3, 169.

23. Malick, A. and Andrew Grant, J. (1997) 'Antihistamines in the treatment of asthma.' *Allergy 52*, Suppl. 34, 55–66.

24. Bruce, C., Weatherstone, R., Seaton, A. and Taylor, W.H. (1976) 'Histamine levels in plasma, blood and urine in severe asthma and the effect of corticosteroid treatment.' *Thorax 31*, 6, 724–729.

25. Oby, E. and Janigro, D. (2006) 'The blood–brain barrier and epilepsy.' *Epilepsia 47*, 11, 1761–1774.

26. Abbott, N.J. (2000) 'Inflammatory mediators and modulation of blood–brain barrier permeability.' *Cell. Mol. Neurobiol. 20*, 2, 131–147.

27. Fogel, W.A., Andrzejewski, W. and Maslinski, C. (1991) 'Brain histamine in rats with hepatic encephalopathy.' *J. Neurochem. 56*, 1, 38–43.

28. Ellis, A.J., Wendon, J.A. and Williams, R. (2000) 'Subclinical seizure activity and prophylactic phenytoin infusion in acute liver failure: a controlled clinical trial.' *Hepatology 32*, 3, 536–541.

29. Mathiak, G., Wening, J.V., Mathiak, M. and Neville, L.F. (1999) 'Serum cholesterol is elevated in patients with Achilles tendon ruptures.' *Arch. Orthop. Trauma Surg. 119*, 5–6.

30. Deadman, P. and Al-Khafaji, M., with Baker, K. (2007) *A Manual of Acupuncture* (2nd edition). Hove: Journal of Chinese Medicine.

Chapter 28

1. Larsen, W.J. (1997) *Essentials of Human Embryology* (2nd edition). New York, NY: Churchill Livingstone.

Chapter 29

1. Ju-Yi, W., and Robertson, J. (2008) *Applied Channel Theory in Chinese Medicine: Wang Ju-Yi's Lectures on Channel Therapeutics.* Seattle, WA: Eastland Press.

Chapter 30

1. Deadman, P. and Al-Khafaji, M., with Baker, K. (2007) *A Manual of Acupuncture* (2nd edition). Hove: Journal of Chinese Medicine.

2. Mathiak, G., Wening, J.V., Mathiak, M. and Neville, L.F. (1999) 'Serum cholesterol is elevated in patients with Achilles tendon ruptures.' *Arch. Orthop. Trauma Surg. 119*, 5–6.

3. Hoff, B. (1983) The Tao of Pooh. London: Penguin Books.

Appendix 3

1. Craig, A.D. (2002) 'How do you feel? Interoception: the sense of the physiological condition of the body.' *Nat. Rev. Neurosci. 3*, 655–666.

2. Sandahl, B., Ulmsten, U. and Andersson, K.E. (1980) 'Local application of ketocaine for treatment of referred pain in primary dysmenorrhea.' *Acta Obstet. Gynecol. Scand. 59*, 3, 259–260.

INDEX